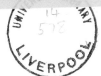

A colour atlas
of
Histology

M.B.L. CRAIGMYLE
MD, MB, ChB
*Senior Lecturer in Histology and Anatomy
University College, Cardiff*

WOLFE MEDICAL PUBLICATIONS LTD
10 Earlham Street   London WC2

Copyright © M B L Craigmyle 1975
Published by Wolfe Medical Publications Ltd 1975
Printed by Smeets-Weert, Holland
SBN 7234 0438 0

General Editor, Wolfe Medical Books
G Barry Carruthers MD (Lond)

Other books in this series already published
A colour atlas of Haematological Cytology
A colour atlas of General Pathology
A colour atlas of Oro-Facial Diseases
A colour atlas of Ophthalmological Diagnosis
A colour atlas of Renal Diseases
A colour atlas of Venereology
A colour atlas of Dermatology
A colour atlas of Infectious Diseases
A colour atlas of Ear, Nose & Throat Diagnosis
A colour atlas of Rheumatology
A colour atlas of Microbiology
A colour atlas of Forensic Pathology
A colour atlas of Paediatrics

Further titles now in preparation
A colour atlas of General Surgical Diagnosis
A colour atlas of Gynaecology
A colour atlas of Clinical Cardiology & Cardiac Pathology
A colour atlas of Physical Signs in Clinical Medicine
A colour atlas of Gastro-Intestinal Endoscopy
A colour atlas of Tropical Medicine & Parasitology
A colour atlas of Orthopaedics
A colour atlas of the Liver
A colour atlas of Respiratory Diseases
A colour atlas of Endocrinology
A colour atlas of Cytology
A colour atlas of Bone Diseases
A colour atlas of Tumour Pathology
A colour atlas of Mycopathology
A colour atlas of Accident Surgery
A colour atlas of Urology
A colour atlas of Staining Techniques
A colour atlas of Dentistry
A colour atlas of Surgical Repair of Jaw Deformities
A colour atlas of Periodontology
A colour atlas of Children's Dentistry

Contents

Preface

Whilst this book has been aimed primarily at undergraduate students of medicine and dentistry, it should have a wide appeal for postgraduate members of both professions attempting Primary Fellowship examinations. I hope, further, that the book will fill a void in the bookshelves of undergraduates reading biological sciences such as zoology, physiology, microbiology, biochemistry, human biology and nursing.

The book represents a record of the appearance, under the light microscope, of the tissues, organs and systems of the human body. (To illustrate a particular point tissue from a species other than man has sometimes been used.) Advances in knowledge stemming from electron microscopic studies have been included in the text, although no electron micrographs themselves are printed as this would have made the book too unwieldy. When reference to the magnification of a picture is made, the following code applies: 'low power' is from ×25 to ×50; 'medium power' from ×100 to ×200; and 'high power' from ×250 to ×600. The abbreviations *TS* and *LS* in the captions refer to 'transverse section' and 'longitudinal section'.

For 15 years I sat at the feet of Professor Fritz Jacoby and during that time he was never unwilling to give me of his time and energy to pass on his profound knowledge of histology. He also supplied some of the preparations from which the book is illustrated. To him I owe a substantial debt of gratitude, therefore. I should also like to thank Professor J D Lever, Head of the Department of Anatomy, University College, Cardiff for allowing me to use some of the demonstration and class slides in the departmental collection. To Professor R E Coupland of the Department of Human Morphology, University of Nottingham I am indebted for the preparation illustrated in figure **192**. Figures **134**, **212** and **501** were taken from preparations given me by Professor D B Moffat of the Department of Anatomy, University College, Cardiff. Dr A J Dark, Department of Ophthalmology, University of Sheffield supplied the preparation illustrated in figures **514–519**. Finally I should like to thank Mr L Jones, Chief Technician, Department of Anatomy, University College, Cardiff who over twenty years cut and stained, as only he can, much of my own material. Miss Pamela Lee and Miss Gail Lightfoot typed the manuscript, and to them I am indebted. Finally, I wish to thank my wife for her constant encouragement and uncomplaining sacrifice without which the book would never have come to fruition.

Staining methods

Most of the information concerning the effect of dyes on tissues has been obtained empirically. The purpose of a staining method is to render conspicuous the various components of a tissue so that they may be observed. However, one element alone in a tissue, e.g. an elastic fibre, may be stained selectively whilst all others remain unstained. Dyes may be artificial or naturally occurring.

With relatively few exceptions the preparations illustrated in this book have been stained by one of the four methods shown opposite, all of which bring out nucleus and cytoplasm in contrasting colours and also, with the exception of H & E, cytoplasm and collagen, which are commonly adjacent.

Differential staining is brought about by the fact that tissue components may be acidic, basic or amphoteric—i.e. the p.H. of the fluid in which they are immersed causes their electric charge to vary. All dyes form ionic solutions, some being positively and others negatively charged. Usually cationic (basic) dyes stain acidic tissue components whereas anionic (acidic) dyes do the reverse. Some dyes such as haematin are amphoteric, being basic in certain p.H. ranges and acidic in others.

Staining methods other than those shown opposite are employed when the degree of differential staining required is not achieved by any one of these methods. A sizeable number of such stains have been used but it is beyond the scope of this brief synopsis to enumerate the ingredients employed in each.

1 *Iron Haematoxylin and Picrofuchsin (Van Gieson)*
Nuclei—brown.
Cytoplasm—yellow.
Collagen—red.

2 *Azocarmine and Aniline Blue (Azan, or Mallory's Stain)*
Nuclei—red.
Cytoplasm—purple-grey.
Collagen—blue.

3 *Haematoxylin and Orange G-Erythrosin (H & OGE)*
Nuclei—purple.
Cytoplasm—pink.
Collagen—orange.

4 *Haematoxylin and Eosin (H & E)*
Nuclei—purple.
Cytoplasm—pink.
Collagen—pink.

1

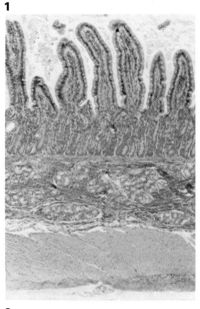

2

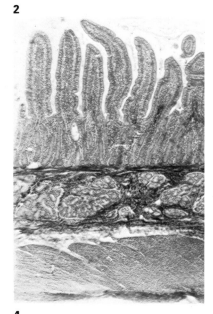

3

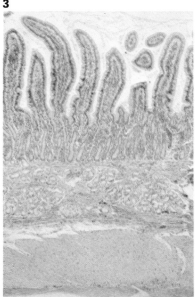

4

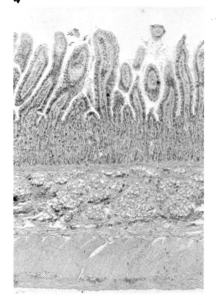

Epithelium

Epithelium is one of four basic tissues of the body; the others are connective, muscular and nervous tissues. The majority of epithelia are composed of closely-packed cells with little by way of intercellular substance between them. Epithelium occurs either as a protective covering or in the form of glands. All epithelia are separated by a basement membrane from the connective tissue which is always adjacent. Where epithelium forms a covering layer, it may be simple or compound: in simple (and pseudo-stratified) epithelium each and every cell is in contact with the basement membrane, whereas in compound epithelia the cells are stacked and the deep cells alone rest on the basement membrane.

Classification of epithelia

Simple
Squamous
Cubical
Columnar
Pseudo-stratified columnar

Compound
Transitional
Stratified squamous
    mucous membrane variety
    skin variety (= epidermis)
Stratified cubical
Stratified columnar

Atypical
Thymus
Stellate reticulum of enamel organ
    of developing tooth
Stratified squamous epithelium
    overlying the lymphoid tissue
    of oro-pharyngeal isthmus

Glandular
Exocrine
Endocrine

All the glands in the body are composed of epithelial cells. A gland whose secretion is liberated onto a body surface, either internal or external, is designated as being an exocrine gland; the epithelial cells forming the secretory parts (and the duct portions when present) of such a gland will be arranged in the form of a sheet of lining cells. A gland which discharges its secretion into the blood stream is called an endocrine gland and such glands are mere clumps of epithelial cells which are not connected with any surface of the body, internal or external.

Exemptions to the generalisation that epithelium is composed of closely-packed cells are few. However, in the thymus, in the stellate reticulum of the enamel organ of the developing tooth and in the lining epithelium of certain parts of the mouth and pharynx (e.g. tonsil and adenoids) are to be found examples of epithelia in which the cells are separated by connective tissue elements in varying degree: such epithelia are designated atypical (reticulated) epithelia. Further information on them will be found in the appropriate chapters.

Basement membrane
The basement membrane separating epithelium from connective tissues varies in its degree of development with the type of epithelium: it is poorly seen in transitional epithelium but marked in epidermis. It is homogeneous in appearance when examined by the light or the electron microscope. It is composed of fine reticular fibres bathed in a gel of mucopolysaccharide ground substance. It can be stained by methods for reticular fibres (e.g. silver impregnation) or by methods for mucopolysaccharides (e.g. the periodic acid—Schiff reaction).

Mucous membrane
All epithelia (except the epidermis of the skin) are normally moist and form one of the constituents of a mucous membrane, which is the moist inner lining of all viscera. The other constant component of a mucous membrane is the areolar connective tissue (the corium or lamina propria) underneath the epithelium. In the case of the mucosa of the alimentary canal, there is a third constituent present, namely a layer of smooth muscle (muscularis mucosae).

Myoepithelium
All undifferentiated cells possess the properties of motility, contractility and conductivity. The ability to contract is retained into the adult differentiated state by certain epithelial cells known as myoepithelial cells. These cells are found in contact with the basement membrane of the terminal tubules of certain glands (e.g. sweat glands). Myoepithelial cells are stellate in outline and send processes round the terminal tubule of the gland: they possess cytoplasmic myofilaments which resemble closely those seen in smooth muscle cells. Myoepithelial cells are presumed to be contractile, therefore, and by their contraction would cause the secretory product of the gland to be liberated from the cytoplasm of the lining cells into the lumen. Because of their position between the basement membrane and the gland cells, myoepithelial cells are thought to be active also in the transfer of nutrients to the latter.

Exocrine glands
These may be unicellular or multicellular. The goblet cells in the epithelia of the alimentary and respiratory tracts represent examples of unicellular glands. Multicellular glands may be composed exclusively of secretory cells and such glands will not have ducts. In the majority of glands however, only the deepest cells secrete, and the products of the gland reach the surface through the intermediary of a duct system. Multicellular glands may be simple (unbranched) or compound (branched).

Junctional complexes in epithelium
Under the light microscope, dark bands known as terminal bars are seen between the apices of columnar epithelial cells where they abut on a lumen.

With the electron microscope this structure is seen more clearly and has been called a junctional complex, which has three components:

A tight junction. This is juxtaluminal in location and extends around the entire apical circumference of the cell. The outer leaflet of the plasma membrane blends with the outer leaflet of the membrane of adjacent cells so that the extracellular space is obliterated. A complete seal between the lumen and the extracellular space is thus brought about.

A loose junction. Here the extracellular space is of normal proportions but intracellular plaques of filamentous material are found. The function of this component of the complex is obscure.

A desmosome. This constitutes the third and deepest part of the complex and appears to be an attachment device between the cells.

---

5 *Simple squamous epithelium (H & E)* Ceruminous gland of the external auditory meatus.

6 *Simple cubical epithelium (H & E)* Amniotic surface of placenta.

7 *Simple columnar epithelium (H & E)* Alveolus of prostate gland.

8 *Pseudo-stratified columnar epithelium (H & E)* Vas deferens.

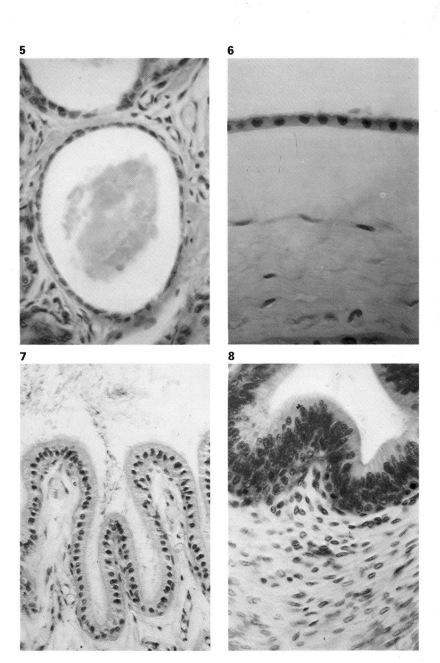

9 *Simple columnar epithelium with a striated (brush) border (H & E)* Small intestine. The brush border at this magnification appears as a dark pink homogeneous line. A single pale goblet cell is seen (centre). The very dark nuclei belong to lymphocytes migrating through the epithelium.

10 *Pseudo-stratified ciliated columnar epithelium (H & E)* Trachea. The cilia appear as a fringe at the surface. Several rows of nuclei are present, but every cell rests on the basement membrane.

11 *Compound epithelium, transitional epithelium (H & E)* Urinary bladder. The cells of the surface (cuticular) layer are umbrella-shaped. The cells of the middle layer are pear-shaped and the cells of the basal layer are columnar.

9

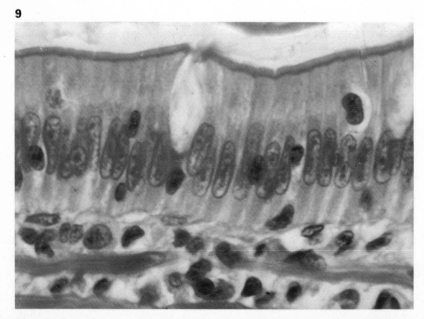

10

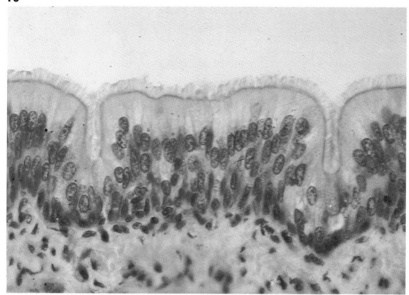

11

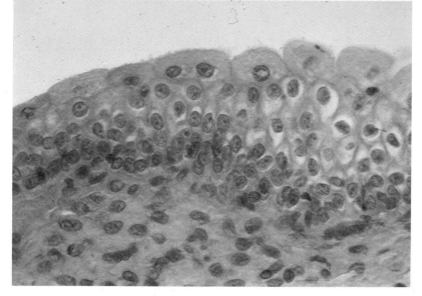

12 *Compound epithelium, thick skin (H & E)* The epidermis exhibits five strata from deep to superficial. These are:

A, stratum germinitivum. A single row of columnar cells.

B, stratum spinosum. Exhibits several rows of cells, the deepest of which are polyhedral and the most superficial of which are squamous. All possess spines or prickles round their circumference. These cytoplasmic projections are not visible at this magnification however.

C, stratum granulosum. This is composed of two or three rows of squamous cells whose cytoplasm is packed with granules of keratohyalin and which are stained dark purple.

D, stratum lucidum. This is composed of two or three layers of squamous anucleate cells whose outlines are indistinct, and the stratum appears as a structureless pale zone. This stratum is often absent (see **14**).

E, stratum corneum. This multi-layered zone of anucleate squames is the major component of thick skin from regions such as the palms and soles. It is not shown in its entirety in the photograph. The duct of a sweat gland can be seen coiling through it.

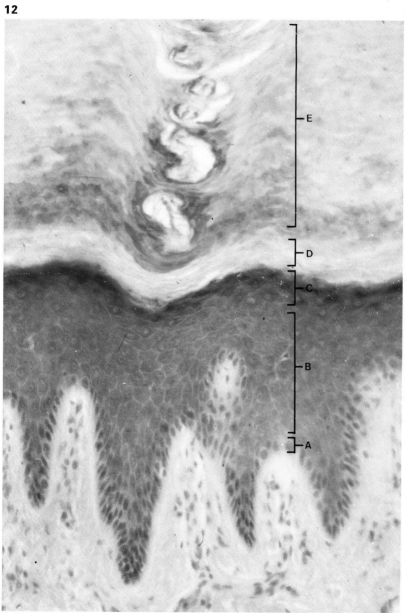

13 *Compound epithelium, stratified squamous epithelium of the mucous membrane variety (H & E)* Tongue. The basal layer (stratum germinitivum) is a single row of columnar cells. The stratum spinosum (prickle cell layer) is multilayered and the cells range from polyhedral (deep) to squamous (superficial).

14 *Compound epithelium, thick skin (H & E)* The stratum lucidum, as here, is often absent in thick skin.

15 *Compound epithelium, thin skin (H & E)* In thin skin the stratum lucidum is always absent and the stratum corneum is poorly developed.

16 *Compound epithelium, stratified cubical epithelium (H & E)* Lactiferous duct of breast showing a stratified epithelium in which the surface cells are cubical.

17 *Compound epithelium, stratified columnar epithelium (H & E)* Section of a salivary duct showing a stratified epithelium in which the superficial cells are columnar.

13

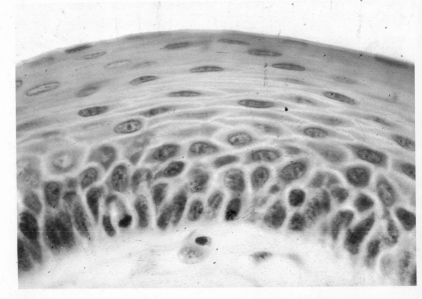

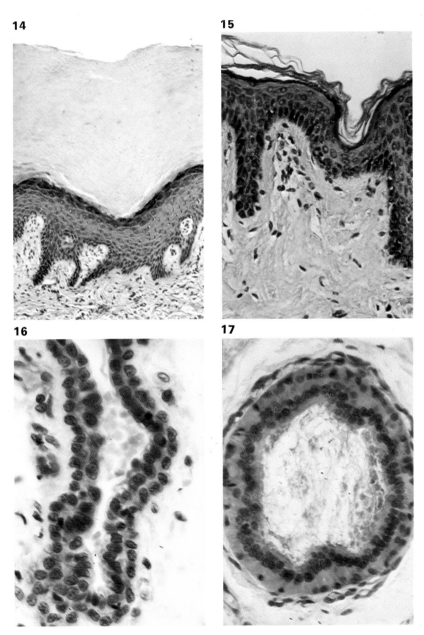

18 *Basement membrane, stratified squamous epithelium of epiglottis (Silver and PAS)* The reticular fibre component has been demonstrated by silver impregnation, and the mucopolysaccharide content is stained pink by the PAS reaction.

19 *Basement membrane, glomerulus of kidney (Silver and PAS)* As **18**.

20 *Myoepithelium 'apocrine' sweat gland (H & E)* The foot processes of the cell appear as a row of dots just inside the basement membrane.

21 *Myoepithelium, sweat gland (PAS reaction)* The cell processes are here cut longitudinally and appear as pink slashes.

22 *Myoepithelium, sweat gland (Silver)* The myoepithelial cell processes appear as dark slashes.

23 *Myoepithelium, submaxillary gland (Alkaline phosphatase reaction)* A myoepithelial cell is seen in profile view at the bottom of the picture.

18

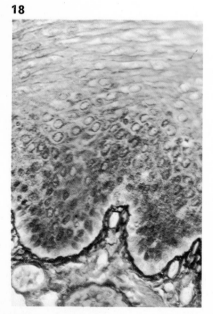

19

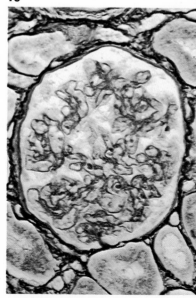

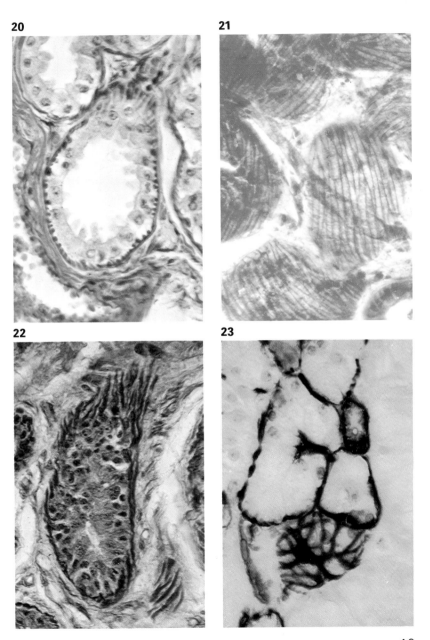

24 *Atypical epithelium (H & E)* The stratified squamous epithelium of the tonsil is heavily infiltrated with lymphocytes.

25 *Atypical epithelium (H & E)* The stellate reticulum of the enamel organ of the developing tooth is so named because the epithelial cells are star-shaped, being separated by large amounts of intercellular substance.

26 *Simple test tube gland, body of uterus (H & E)*

27 *Simple alveolar gland, sebaceous gland (H & E)*

28 *Compound tubular gland, cervix of uterus (H & E)*

29 *Compound tubulo-alveolar gland, mammary gland (H & E)*

24

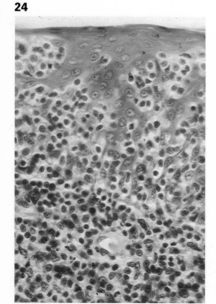

25

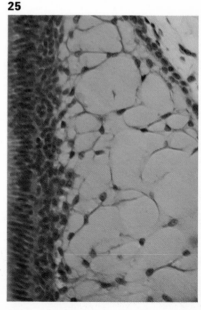

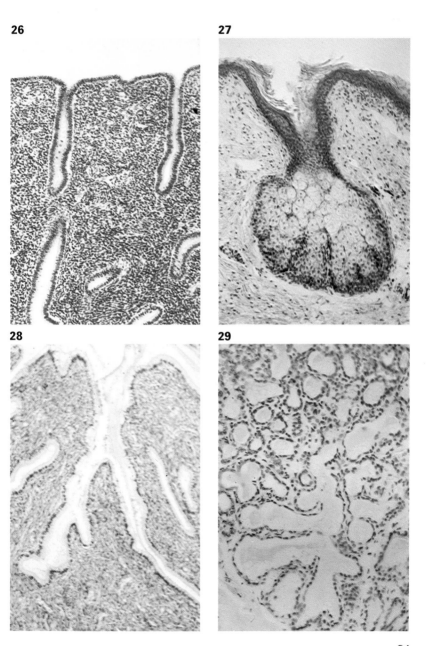

Connective Tissue

In contrast to epithelium, in which intercellular substance is negligible in quantity, connective tissue is characterised by an excess of intercellular material over cells. The physical attributes of all connective tissues except adipose tissue are directly attributable to the nature of the ground substance: in blood, for example, the intercellular substance is fluid whereas in bone it is rock hard. In adipose tissue, however, it is *intracellular* fat which confers on this tissue its specific properties. It must not be inferred from what has been said, however, that connective tissue cells are unimportant; they serve to produce and maintain the intercellular substance. In some connective tissues (e.g. bone) only one cell type is present whereas in others (e.g. areolar tissue) many different kinds of cell occur. The intercellular material consists of a sol or gel complex of protein and mucopolysaccharide which bathes the fibres: these are of three types—collagen, elastic and reticular.

Classification of connective tissues

Loose
Areolar tissue
Reticular tissue
Adipose tissue
Blood

Dense
unformed
Dermis of skin
Submucosa of viscera
formed
Tendon
Ligament
Aponeurosis
Elastic ligament

formed, continued
Cartilage
  hyaline
  yellow elastic
  white fibrous
Bone
  cancellous
  compact
Dentine

Collagen fibres

These 'white' fibres are in fact colourless but appear white when packed in bundles. The bundles of fibres branch but the individual component collagen fibres do not. Collagen fibres possess great tensile strength and are composed of the protein collagen which has a molecular weight of 340,000 and a size of 2,900Å × 140Å. The fibres are formed by cells called fibroblasts: they stain pink with eosin, blue with Mallory's stain, and red with Van Gieson's stain.

Elastic fibres

These fibres are yellow in colour, homogeneous in appearance and vary greatly in diameter. They exhibit branching and are composed of the albuminoid protein elastin. They can be stained selectively even if not specifically by a number of dyes such as resorcin-fuchsin, orcein or aldehyde-fuchsin. They are produced by connective tissue cells and specifically by fibroblasts in all probability.

Reticular (argyrophil) fibres
These are thought by some authorities to be identical with collagen fibres and by others to be different. They are of finer diameter than collagen fibres, they branch and they can, unlike collagen, be impregnated by silver. They appear to merge with collagen bundles. Reticular fibres form the framework of organs such as lymph nodes, spleen, liver, and kidneys and are found around smooth muscle fibres. They are not found in areolar tissue as a rule. Where loose connective tissue has a complement of such fibres, as in the lamina propria of the gut, it is called reticular tissue.

Endothelium
Every connective tissue space is lined by flattened connective tissue cells known as endothelial cells. This endothelial lining is very difficult to distinguish from simple squamous epithelium. A lining of endothelium is found in the following situations:

Blood vessels	*Peritoneal cavity*
Chambers of the heart	*Pericardial cavity*
Lymph vessels	*Anterior chamber of the eye*
Pleural cavity	*Bony labyrinth of the inner ear*

Areolar tissue
This tissue is of widespread occurrence in the body as the packing material between the organs; it also forms an investment for muscles, blood vessels and nerves. It is composed of elastic and collagen fibres embedded in ground substance and nine different cell types occur: fibroblasts, macrophages, fat cells, mast cells, pigment cells, plasma cells, lymphocytes, eosinophils and undifferentiated mesenchymal cells.

Adipose tissue
This tissue is also of widespread occurrence since it comprises the subcutaneous connective tissue and forms the capsule of some organs. It is composed exclusively of fat cells with a film of areolar tissue surrounding each. It functions as a food reserve, a thermal insulator and a mechanical buffer.

Tendon, ligament and aponeurosis
These tissues are composed of (primary) collagenous bundles running in

parallel, and fibroblasts. Areolar tissue separates each large (secondary) bundle. They have a scant blood supply.

Elastic ligament
Such structures as the ligamentum nuchae are composed of greatly enlarged branching elastic fibres separated by areolar tissue.

Cartilage
This occurs in three forms, hyaline, yellow elastic and white fibrous: of these, the first two have rather similar physical properties inasmuch as they are pliable and fairly hard, whereas white fibrocartilage has physical properties akin to those of tendon. Hyaline and elastic cartilage have a close resemblance histologically. Each is enclosed in a perichondrium of dense fibrous tissue. The cartilage cells lie singly or in groups (chondrones) in a hyaline matrix. This matrix is composed of a gel of mucopolysaccharide (chondroitin sulphuric acid) within which are embedded collagen and elastic fibres in the case of elastic cartilage and collagen fibres alone in the case of hyaline cartilage. The fibres are invisible, however, because their refractive index is the same as that of the ground substance. Hyaline and elastic cartilage are both avascular. White fibrocartilage is composed of collagen bundles with rows of chondrocytes between.

Bone
Bone is found in two forms, cancellous and compact. Cancellous bone is avascular, and compact bone is not. Both consist of bone cells or osteocytes lying singly in spaces known as lacunae, in the homogeneous matrix. The matrix is permeated by fine canaliculi linking adjacent lacunae and occupied by cytoplasmic processes of the osteocytes: these canaliculi permit of diffusion of nutrients through the bone substance. The matrix is composed of collagen fibres embedded in a calcified ground substance. In compact bone the ground

continued

---

30 *Areolar connective tissue (Verhoeff's elastic)* The cell nuclei are pink. Elastic fibres are fine purple lines. Collagen bundles appear as broad pink bands.

31 *Areolar connective tissue (Brazilin)* Cell nuclei are brown. The elastic fibres appear as fine brown lines and the collagen bundles as broad brown bands.

32 *Areolar connective tissue (Silver)* Silver impregnation of the ground substance stains it dark brown. The areas occupied by the cells are unstained.

33 *Pigmented areolar connective tissue (H & E)* Many irregular melanin-containing chromatophores are seen.

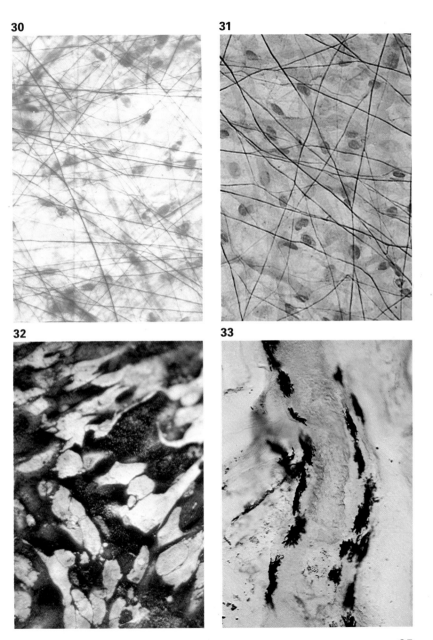

30

31

32

33

25

substance is disposed in layers or lamellae which are arranged in concentric fashion with respect to a large (Haversian) canal containing an arteriole, a venule and nerves. In the angles between these (Haversian) lamellae are to be found interstitial lamellae arranged irregularly. The osteocytes lie in concentric rows between the lamellae. The Haversian canal with its contained blood vessels and associated lamellae and osteocytes collectively constitute a Haversian system. Each system is surrounded by an area of dense matrix known as a cementing line which separates it from adjacent systems. Nutrition diffuses from the Haversian vessels to the periphery of the system, and to facilitate this there are always more canaliculi on the inside of a lacuna than on its outside: indeed the most circumferential lacunae have canaliculi on their inner aspect only.

---

34 *Areolar connective tissue (H & E)* There is an accumulation of lymphocytes and plasma cells: the latter are characterised by an eccentric nucleus and abundant bright pink cytoplasm.

35 *Areolar connective tissue (PAS reaction)* Several mast cells can be seen.

36 *Areolar connective tissue (Sudan IV)* A small cluster of fat cells and a nerve can be seen.

37 *Adipose tissue (H & E)* The tissue is composed in large measure of fat cells whose fat globule has been dissolved during preparation and they appear as empty ghosts.

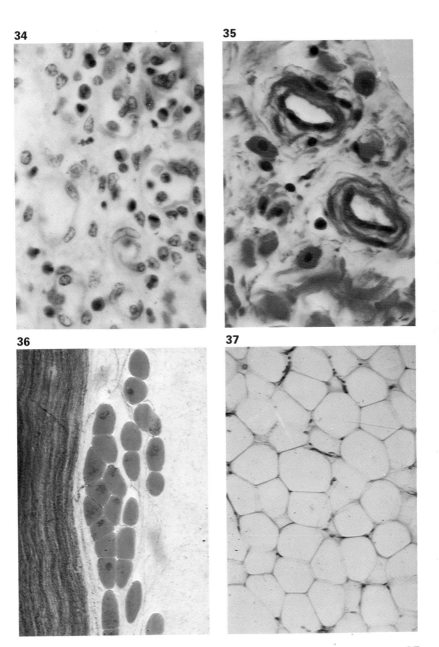

34

35

36

37

27

38 *Endothelium (H & E)* Chest wall showing the parietal pleura. The endothelial nuclei appear as conspicuous surface bulges.

39 *Endothelium (H & E)* Muscular artery. The endothelial cells lining the vessel are clearly delineated.

40 *Endothelium (Silver)* Whole mount of mesentery of the small gut. On one face the endothelial cells have a very irregular outline.

41 *Endothelium (Silver)* The same portion of mesentery shown in **40** at a different focal level. At the opposite face, the endothelial cells have a regularly polyhedral outline.

42 *TS tendon (H & E)* Bundles of dense collagen with star-shaped fibroblast nuclei between are seen.

43 *TS tendon (H & E)* Portions of two secondary bundles of collagen are shown: each secondary bundle is composed in turn of smaller primary collagenous bundles. The fibroblast nuclei are stellate.

38

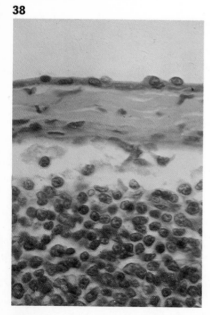

39

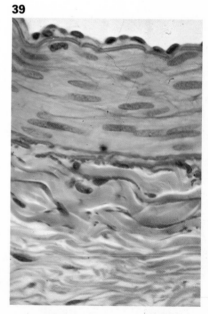

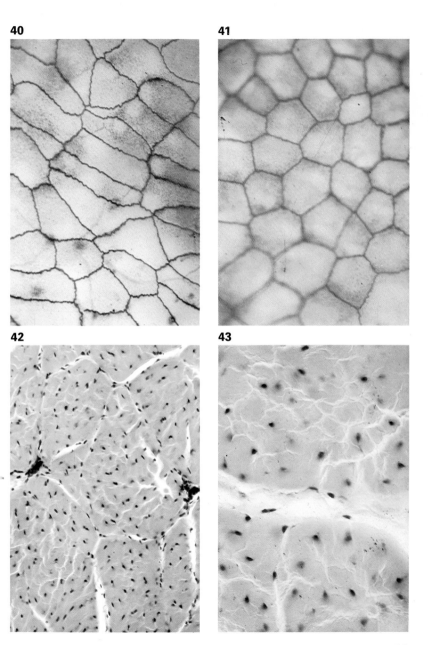

44 *LS tendon (H & E)* Three secondary bundles separated by areolar tissue.

45 *LS tendon (H & E)* Portions of two secondary bundles are seen, with areolar tissue between. Each secondary bundle is subdivisible into smaller primary bundles with elongated fibroblast nuclei between.

46 *TS yellow elastic ligament (Van Gieson)* The elastic fibres are stained yellow, are of large diameter and are surrounded by areolar tissue (stained orange).

47 *TS yellow elastic ligament (H & E)* The elastic fibres are of a homogeneous pink colour. Between them is areolar tissue with fibroblast nuclei.

48 *LS yellow elastic ligament (Van Gieson)* The elastic fibres are stained yellow and the collagen fibres red.

49 *LS yellow elastic ligament (H & E)* The homogeneous elastic fibres branch freely. They are invested by areolar tissue, the fibroblast nuclei of which stain darkly.

44

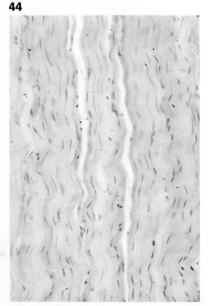

45

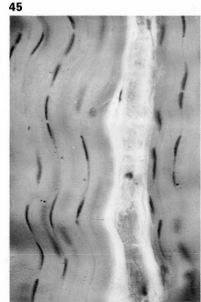

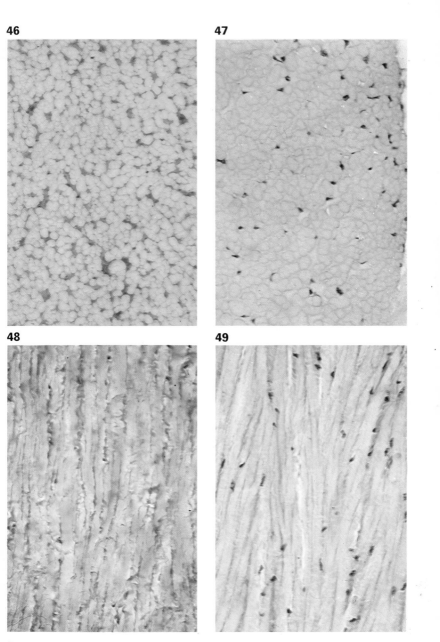

31

50 *Hyaline cartilage, costal cartilage (H & E)* The fibrous perichondrium is at the top; below are flattened chondroblasts. The mature chondrocytes (bottom) lie in groups (chondrones) separated by hyaline matrix.

51 *Elastic cartilage, external auditory meatus (H & E)* At the top is the perichondrium with fibroblasts; below are flattened chondroblasts. The mature chondrocytes (bottom) are separated by matrix which is of hyaline appearance.

52 *Elastic cartilage, epiglottis (Verhoeff's elastic)* The branching elastic fibres can now be seen ramifying around the cartilage cells.

53 *White fibrocartilage, insertion of supraspinatus tendon (H & E)* The collagen bundles are separated by rows of chondrocytes.

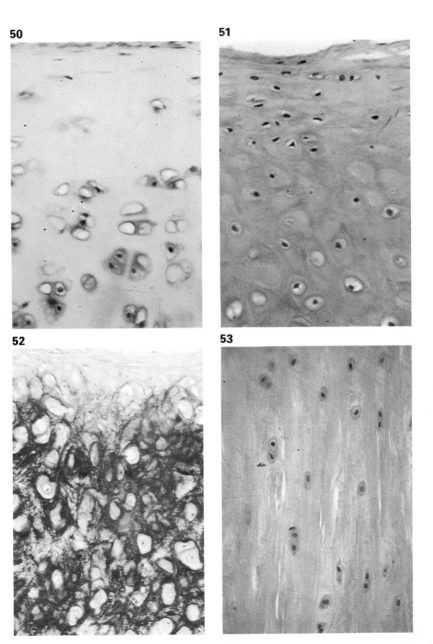

50

51

52

53

33

54 *Cancellous bone (H & E)* The spicules of bone are separated by yellow marrow (adipose tissue).

55 *Cancellous bone (H & E)* High power view of a field from the previous figure. The osteocytes (bone cells) are scattered in the homogeneous bone matrix.

56 *TS compact bone (H & E)* The Haversian systems are clearly to be seen. The osteocytes and bony lamellae are arranged concentrically.

57 *TS compact bone (Schmorl's stain)* The cementing lines surrounding each Haversian system are clearly delineated.

58 *LS compact bone (H & E)*

59 *LS compact bone (Schmorl's stain)*

54

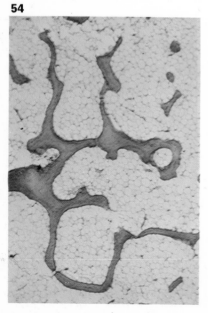

55

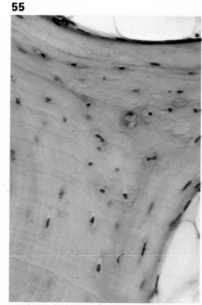

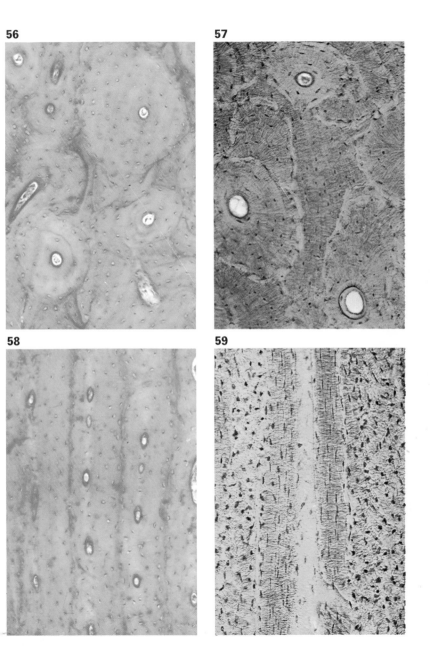

60 *Compact bone (H & E)* High power view of a field from **56**.

61 *Compact bone (Schmorl's stain)* High power view of a field from **57**. The canaliculi radiating from the lacunae are demonstrated.

62 *LS compact bone (H & E)* The Haversian canals branch and anastomose freely.

63 *Sharpey's fibres (H & E)* Supraspinatus insertion. The collagen fibres of the tendon pass into the bone and are known as the fibres of Sharpey.

60

61

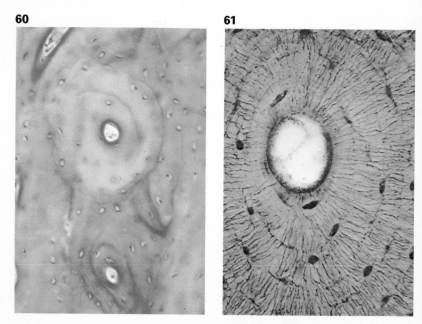

62

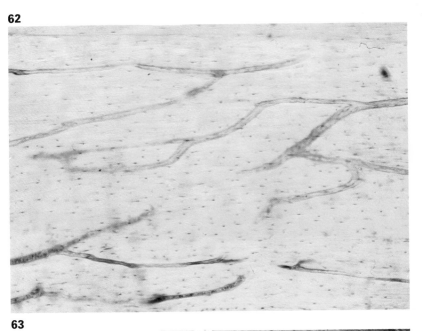

63

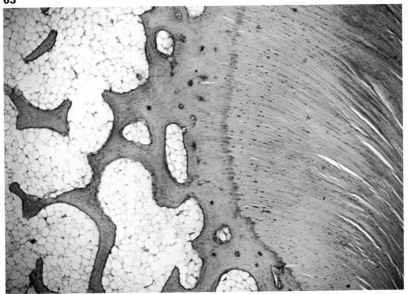

Muscular Tissue

Muscle cells are usually referred to as muscle fibres because invariably they are elongated in one axis. Running in the long axis of the cell are extended contractile elements known as myofibrils: these impart a longitudinal striation to all muscle cells. The myofibrils of some types of muscle cell consist of alternate light and dark bands: the myofibril bands are in register in that the light bands lie opposite one another and the dark bands do likewise. As a result a cross-striation is imparted to the fibre, which is then described as being striated (striped). Muscle is classified histologically according to whether it is cross-striated or not.

Classification of muscle

Smooth or non-striated

Striated
Skeletal muscle
Cardiac muscle

The plasma membrane of a muscle fibre is known as the sarcolemma and it differs in its degree of development from one type of muscle to another. The cytoplasm of a muscle fibre is called sarcoplasm. The sarcoplasm of muscle fibres of all three types is rich in mitochondria. Smooth endoplasmic reticulum, called the sarcoplasmic reticulum, is abundant in both skeletal and cardiac muscle fibres. The fibrous proteins actin and myosin can be extracted from muscle fibres of all types.

Smooth muscle

Muscle of this type is of widespread occurrence being found in the wall of most hollow viscera and of every artery and vein. The fibres vary in length, the shortest (20μ) fibres being found in the wall of arterioles and the longest (500μ) in the myometrium of the pregnant uterus. The fibres taper at each extremity and are about 5μ wide in their central nucleated region. In longitudinal section the nucleus is an elongated ovoid in a relaxed fibre and corkscrew-shaped in a contracted fibre. A transverse section of the fibre usually avoids the nucleus: when sectioned, the latter is of circular outline.

The sarcolemma of smooth muscle is difficult to resolve with the light microscope. Under the electron microscope, there is seen to be a layer of material outside the sarcolemma which resembles closely the basement membrane of epithelium. In Haematoxylin and Eosin preparations smooth muscle fibres are seen to be separated by wide clear (i.e. non-staining) areas: these can be stained by the periodic acid—Schiff method indicating that they contain ground substance. In sections subjected to silver impregnation, many reticular (argyrophil) fibres can be seen spiralling round the muscle fibre: it is believed that they act as a harness against which the fibre can brace itself in the act of contraction.

Smooth muscle is innervated by the autonomic nervous system but it is not thought that every fibre receives a nerve terminal, but only a proportion do. It is believed that the stimulus to contract is passed from one fibre to the next across regions which resemble closely the tight junctions of epithelia and in which the outer leaflets of the plasma membranes of the adjacent smooth muscle fibres fuse, obliterating the extracellular space.

Skeletal muscle

Skeletal muscle fibres are multinucleate giant cells ranging in length from a few millimetres to a few centimetres and in breadth from 10 to 150 microns. The sarcolemma is distinct; just inside it lie the many oval nuclei, distributed randomly within the fibre. The fibres can be seen when cut in longitudinal section to possess distinct striations both transversely and longitudinally. These are caused by the myofibrils which run lengthwise in the fibre and which are composed of alternating dark anisotropic (A) bands and light isotropic (I) bands. Under oil immersion, a dark (Z) line can be seen running down the centre of the light band and a pale (H) line across the middle of the dark band.

In transverse section, skeletal muscle fibres are seen to be roughly circular in outline and appear stippled due to the cut ends of the myofibrils. The myofibrils may be distributed evenly in the sarcoplasm or may be in clumps—areas of Cohnheim—separated by homogeneous sarcoplasm. One or more nuclei may be seen in a transverse section of a skeletal muscle fibre: the nuclei appear spherical.

Two types of skeletal muscle fibres, red and white, are found in admixture in human skeletal muscle. The red fibre is the majority type: it is of small diameter, is rich in the pigment myoglobin and is relatively lacking in myofibrils. The white fibre is of greater diameter, and has more myofibrils than the red: it has, as a result, a much more pronounced cross-striation. It has a relative lack of myoglobin.

With the electron microscope, the sarcolemma is seen to be a composite of the following entities:

The plasma membrane of the muscle fibre.

A layer of homogeneous basement membrane material (lamina densa or external basal lamina).

A network of fine reticular fibres.

Skeletal muscle fibres are invested by highly vascular areolar tissue containing collagen, elastic and reticular fibres; this is known as the endomysium. The muscle fibres are collected into bundles invested by a sheath of dense connective tissue, the perimysium. The entire muscle is invested by areolar tissue, the muscle sheath or epimysium.

With the electron microscope, the myofibrils are seen to be composed of even finer elements known as myofilaments of which there are two sorts. One type is composed of the protein myosin, is of some 100Å diameter, and is confined to the A band. The other kind is composed of the protein actin, is narrow (50Å) and is attached at one end to the Z line of the I band. The other extremity lies free in the A band.

The innervation of skeletal muscle

Every skeletal muscle fibre has an associated nerve terminal. The cell body of the neurone in question, known as the lower motor neurone, lies in the anterior horn of the spinal cord, and its axon may innervate from 1 to 100 skeletal muscle fibres. The point of contact of nerve terminal and muscle fibre is known as a motor end plate, and here the muscle fibre is swollen and possesses a localised accumulation of nuclei and mitochondria. The nerve axon loses its myelin sheath just before it reaches the muscle fibre: its connective tissue sheath (endoneurium) is continuous with the endomysium. The axon branches and its terminals sink into surface recesses of the muscle fibre, only the amorphous component of the sarcolemma intervening between the plasma membranes of axon and muscle fibre.

The proprioceptive sensory nerve terminals in skeletal muscle are known as muscle spindles. These are encapsulated collections of attenuated modified skeletal muscle fibres and their associated nerve. There are generally about half a dozen muscle fibres in the spindle, each being a few millimetres long and attached by its extremities to endomysium or tendon. Sensory nerves arborise round the central region of the fibre in spiral fashion.

Cardiac muscle

This is a pseudo-syncytium of branching fibres linked by surface specialisations known as intercalated discs. Myofibrils identical to those found in skeletal muscle occur in cardiac muscle but are less densely packed with the result that the cross-striation of cardiac muscle is less pronounced than is that of skeletal muscle.

In longitudinal section, the fibres of cardiac muscle are seen to branch and interconnect and to have oval nuclei located centrally. Dark lines known as intercalated discs can be seen running transversely across the fibre in suitably stained preparations. These do not usually run a straight course but cross the

continued

---

64 *LS smooth muscle (H & OGE)* The fibres are elongated and have oval nuclei centrally located. Longitudinal striations alone are present.

65 *TS smooth muscle (H & E)* The fibres, and their nuclei when sectioned, are circular in outline. Note the clear halo around each fibre where the (unstained) reticular fibres lie.

64

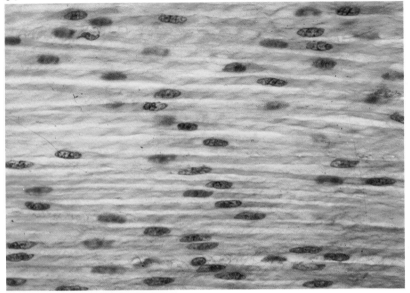

65

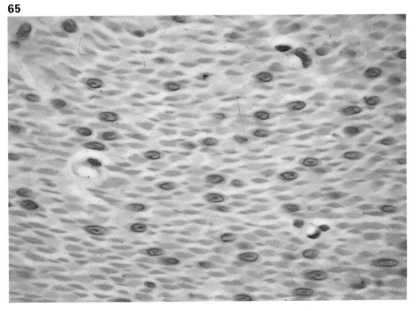

fibre in step fashion. They represent the interval between adjacent muscle fibres and present, under the electron microscope, three different regions comparable to the tight junction, loose junction and desmosome of the junctional complex of epithelium. The myofibrils diverge to pass either side of the nucleus with the result that a region of clear sarcoplasm lies at each nuclear pole: here the brown pigment lipofuscin progressively accumulates with age. Abundant mitochondria occur at the poles of the nucleus, in addition.

In transverse section, the fibres are seen to be of irregular size and outline, with central nuclei of spherical shape. The sarcoplasm has a granular appearance as in skeletal muscle, and the myofibrils may or may not be grouped into areas of Cohnheim.

Cardiac muscle fibres are invested by highly vascular loose connective tissue containing many reticular and a few collagen fibres. The connective tissue elements are not organised into endomysium, perimysium and epimysium as in skeletal muscle, however.

Impulse-conducting fibres

Some cardiac muscle fibres are specialised for impulse conduction rather than contraction. These so-called Purkinje fibres are found in the atrioventricular bundle (of His) and are of larger diameter than contractile cardiac muscle fibres. They are characterised further by the fact that they possess myofibrils only at the periphery of the fibres, so that the nucleus is surrounded by a halo of clear sarcoplasm. Purkinje fibres exhibit intercalated discs and are commonly binucleate. They are continuous eventually with ordinary contractile cardiac muscle.

Nerve supply of cardiac muscle

Autonomic fibres of both sympathetic and parasympathetic origin pass to cardiac muscle, but motor end plates are not encountered. Non-myelinated nerve terminals with synaptic vesicles can be seen in close relation to cardiac muscle fibres under the electron microscope.

---

66 *TS and LS smooth muscle (Silver)* Wall of small intestine. In the upper half of the field is the inner circular coat with the outer longitudinal coat below. The reticular fibre investment is stained black.

67 *LS smooth muscle (Silver)* This high power field from **66** shows the reticular fibres spiralling around the muscle fibres.

66

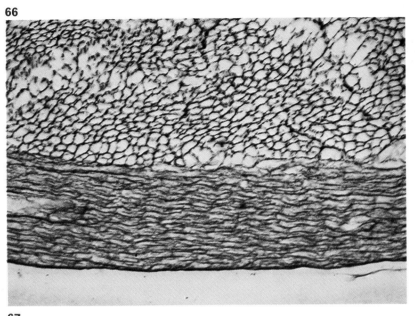

67

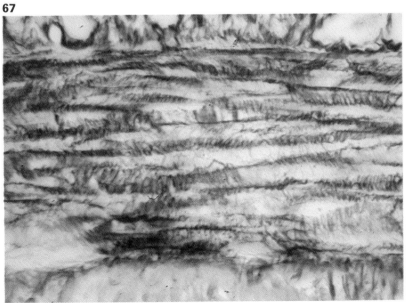

68 *TS skeletal muscle (H & E)* The fibres are circular in outline. The nuclei lie at the periphery of the fibre. The sarcoplasm is here homogeneous.

69 *LS skeletal muscle (H & E)* The fibres are multinucleate. The cross-striations are not demonstrated well by this stain.

70 *LS skeletal muscle (Masson)* The cross-striations can be seen clearly. Collagen is stained green.

71 *LS skeletal muscle (Silver)* The cross-striations are again well demonstrated.

68

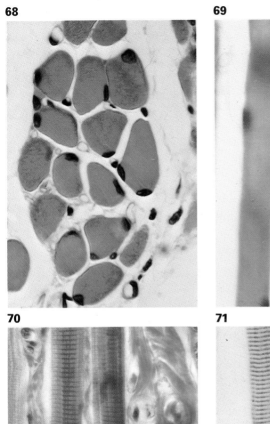

69

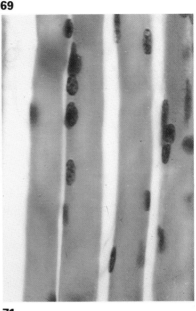

70

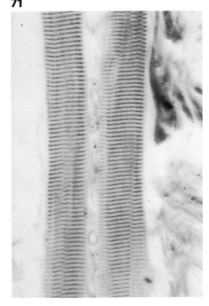

71

45

72 *Motor end plates in skeletal muscle (Silver)* Several motor end plates can be seen as dark areas. A branch of the nerve passes to each.

73 *Motor end plate in skeletal muscle (Silver)* The nerve terminal is seen to branch. Several muscle nuclei can be seen.

74 *Skeletal muscle, musculo-tendinous junction (H & E)* The skeletal muscle fibre endings are rounded and the connective tissue of the muscle is continuous with that of the tendon.

72

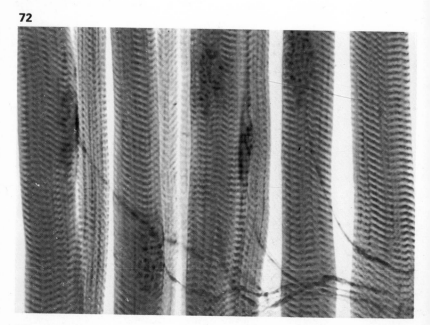

73

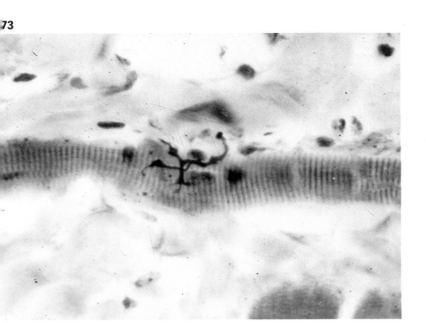

74

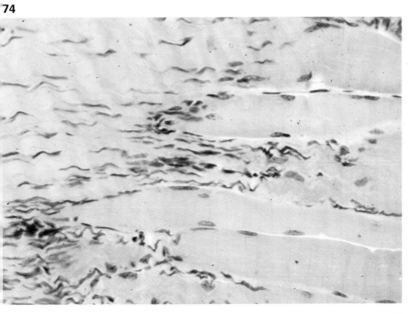

75 *Skeletal muscle, muscle spindle (H & E)* The upper half of the field contains unmodified skeletal muscle. In the lower half of the field the fibres are attenuated and enclosed in a capsule of connective tissue.

76 *Skeletal muscle, muscle spindle (Silver)* This field shows nerve fibres spiralling around the attenuated muscle fibres of a muscle spindle.

77 *LS cardiac muscle (H & E)* In this field the syncytial arrangement of the fibres is seen.

78 *TS cardiac muscle (H & E)* The fibres are of irregular outline and have central nuclei. Many capillaries are present in the adjacent loose connective tissue.

79 *LS cardiac muscle (H & E)* The intercalated discs can be seen as dark bands running across the fibres. The cross-striations are clearly visible.

75

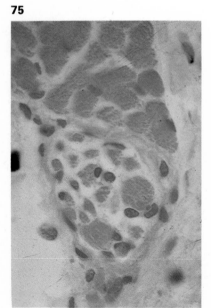

76

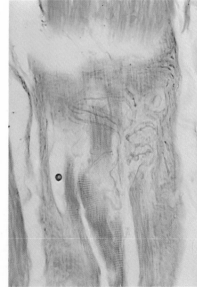

77

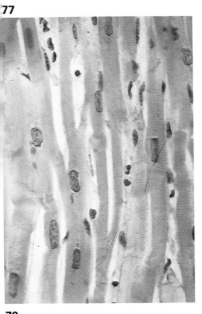

78

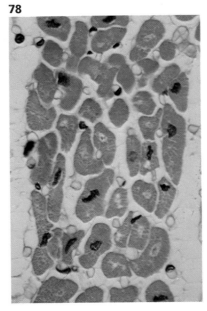

79

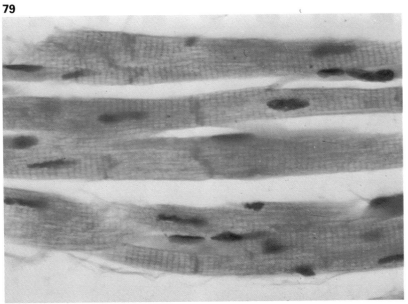

80 *Cardiac muscle, Purkinje fibres (H & E)* The upper half of the field shows unmodified cardiac muscle. At the bottom are the much larger Purkinje fibres.

81 *Cardiac muscle, TS Purkinje fibres (H & E)* These have myofibrils only at the periphery. The centre of the fibres is occupied by the nucleus which is surrounded by clear sarcoplasm.

82 *Cardiac muscle, LS Purkinje fibres (H & E)* The large size of the fibres is again manifest.

83 *Cardiac muscle, Purkinje fibres (Iron haematoxylin)* Unmodified cardiac muscle is seen in TS at the lower left. In the upper centre some Purkinje fibres are seen becoming continuous with this muscle. More Purkinje fibres lie on the right.

80

81

82

83

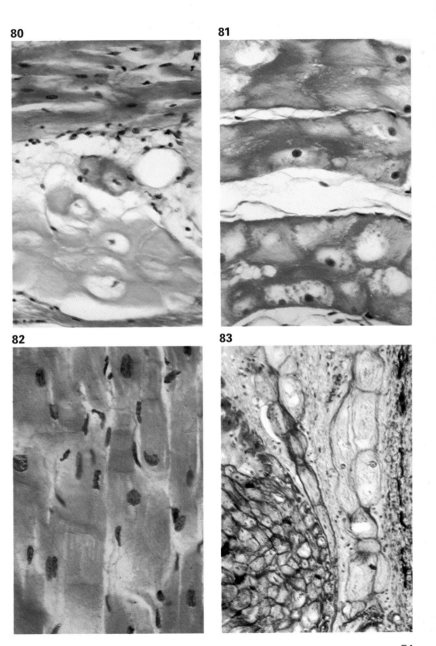

Nervous Tissue

In nervous tissue the cells have adapted specifically so as to be able to transmit impulses from one part of the body to another. This process is rapid and follows circumscribed pathways composed of nerve cells in series passing the impulse from one to another across submicroscopic gaps known as synapses. Every nerve cell possesses at least one very long cytoplasmic process so that the number of units required to transmit the impulse is kept to a minimum. The basic unit of nervous tissue is the neurone—i.e. a nerve cell and all its processes. The great majority of nerve cells possess many processes and are designated therefore as being multipolar: in such nerve cells one process alone conducts the impulse away from the cell body, and is called an axon. All the other processes are known as dendrites because they convey the impulse towards the cell body. Some nerve cells possess but two processes, an axon and a dendrite and are referred to as being bipolar. Finally, some nerve cells may possess a single process of cytoplasm which divides almost immediately, T-fashion, into an axon and a dendrite: such nerve cells are designated as being pseudo-unipolar.

The cell body (or soma or cyton) of a nerve cell is of variable size ($4-140\mu$) and shape. The nucleus is pale and vesicular (nerve cells in the adult do not divide) and is usually located centrally: a single large conspicuous nucleolus is present. The cytoplasm (or perikaryon) is characterised by the presence of Nissl (or chromidial or tigroid) substance which takes the form of patches of basophilia: with the electron microscope the Nissl substance is seen to be composed of rough-surfaced endoplasmic reticulum. Here the enzymes necessary for the transmission process are manufactured. Nissl substance is found in the dendrites but is absent from the axon and the cytoplasm at the origin of the axon (the axon hillock). After silver impregnation, the cytoplasm exhibits a network of fine filaments known as neurofibrils.

The nervous system is the collective name for all the nervous tissue of the body. It is capable, in addition to transmitting impulses, of correlating them and co-ordinating the responses. It can also store information. The nervous system is subdivisible, on the basis of the nature of the supporting tissue, into a central and a peripheral nervous system. The central nervous system is composed of the paired cerebral hemispheres, the olfactory and optic nerves, the retinae, the midbrain, hindbrain (pons, medulla and cerebellum) and the spinal cord. It possesses a non-fibrous (i.e. cellular) supporting tissue which is known as neuroglia and which is peculiar to it. The peripheral nervous system is composed of the nerves of the body (except the olfactory and optic) and their associated ganglia or nerve cell clumps. The peripheral nervous system relies for support on the ordinary connective tissue of the body.

The nerve cell bodies of the central nervous system lie either in the grey matter, or as localised collections in the white matter. The grey matter comprises vast stretches of nerve cells and their supporting neuroglial cells found in the cortices of cerebrum and cerebellum and in the central region of the spinal cord respectively. The white matter is composed of nerve cell processes and their supporting neuroglial cells. The localised collections of nerve cells found in the white matter are usually, but not universally, called nuclei: such collections occur in all parts of the central nervous system except the spinal cord.

Nerve cell groups in the peripheral nervous system on the other hand, are known as ganglia of which there are two types, ganglia of conduction and ganglia of synapse. In the former category are the sensory ganglia of cranial nerves V, VII, IX and X and the dorsal root ganglia of the spinal nerves. The nerve (usually ganglion) cells of these ganglia are of the pseudo-unipolar type. The ganglia of synapse contain multipolar nerve cells and comprise all the ganglia of the autonomic nervous system—i.e. the sympathetic and parasympathetic ganglia. Sympathetic ganglia in general lie close to the central nervous system whereas the parasympathetic ganglia invariably lie considerable distances from the central nervous system. As a result the preganglionic axon or fibre in the sympathetic system is relatively short and the postganglionic fibre comparatively long. The reverse is true of the parasympathetic system.

Every nerve cell body, whether in the central or peripheral nervous system has supporting cells known as satellite cells in its immediate vicinity. The satellite cells of the nerve cell bodies in the central nervous system are neuroglial cells known as oligodendrocytes whereas the satellite cells of the ganglion cell bodies in the peripheral nervous system are modified connective tissue cells.

Axons

Every nerve cell axon whether it lies in the central or the peripheral nervous system has an investment of either oligodendrocytes or connective tissue cells known as Schwann cells as the case may be. The Schwann cell investment of axons in the peripheral nervous system is sometimes called the neurolemma or neurolemmal sheath of Schwann. Where an axon lies partially within the central nervous system and partially in the peripheral nervous system, the nature of its supporting cells will change at the point where it leaves the central nervous system. Each axon is invested, for a part $(0.5-2\mu)$ of its length by a supporting cell of one or other type. Where one supporting cell hands over to the next, there is a small gap known as a node of Ranvier. The degree of intimacy of relationship between the supporting cells and the axon may be either great or small depending on axon size. In the case of axons over 2μ in diameter the supporting cell wraps its plasma membrane round the axon in Swiss-roll fashion to provide it with what is called its myelin sheath. Oligodendrocytes may provide a myelin sheath for several adjacent axons but Schwann cells stand in relationship to axons in the ratio 1:1. In the case of axons under 2μ the supporting cells have several axons lying in superficial recesses of cytoplasm around their circumference, and such axons are described as being non-myelinated. These features are capable of being observed in detail only at the magnifications possible using the electron microscope. However, the myelin sheath, composed as it is of lipid-rich plasma membrane layers can be demonstrated readily with the light microscope after suitable staining for fats. Axons branch infrequently, do so invariably at a node of Ranvier and the side branch (or collateral) comes off at right angles to the main stem. Axons have a more or less uniform diameter throughout their length, are devoid of Nissl substance but possess mitochondria, microtubules and, near their terminations, spherical synaptic vesicles. Axons terminate in three ways:

By forming synapses with either the axons, the dendrites or cell body of another neurone.

By terminating on skeletal muscle fibres.

By terminating on smooth muscle fibres, cardiac muscle, or myoepithelial cells.

Dendrites

Dendrites exhibit rich branching, the branches coming off at acute angles. Dendrites can be seen to taper in size as they are traced away from their cell of origin. Unlike axons, they contain Nissl substance. The dendrites of multipolar and bipolar nerve cells lack an investment of supporting cells. However, the dendrite of the pseudo-unipolar nerve cells located in the ganglia of conduction differ in that they cannot be distinguished from axons since they do not taper and are myelinated by Schwann cells. The dendritic terminals of multi- and bipolar cells make synaptic connections with axons or their collaterals. The dendrite terminals of pseudo-unipolar nerve cells may lose their myelin sheath and become naked (as in epithelium) or may become encapsulated by connective tissue cells and fibres as in the Meissner and Pacinian corpuscles of the skin. Thus input of information to the nervous system takes place via the dendritic terminals of these pseudo-unipolar cells and they receive their information from three sources:

From the superficial tissues of the body: these are called exteroceptive fibres.

From the viscera—interoceptive fibres.

From the joint capsules and ligaments, from tendons and skeletal muscles—the proprioceptive fibres.

Peripheral nerves

These contain afferent (sensory) fibres and efferent (motor) fibres. The afferent fibres are the dendrites of the pseudo-unipolar nerve cells in the dorsal root ganglia of the nerve in question: they may be exteroceptive or proprioceptive in nature. The motor fibres are of two types, somatic efferent and visceral efferent.

The somatic efferent fibres are the heavily myelinated axons of the multipolar nerve cells in the ventral grey horn of the spinal cord. They enter the nerve via its ventral root and terminate on one or more skeletal muscle fibres at a motor end plate. The visceral efferent fibres will be (post-ganglionic) fibres derived from multipolar nerve cells in the sympathetic ganglia: they will be vasomotor (to the smooth muscle of the blood vessels) pilomotor (to the smooth muscle of the hair follicles) or sudomotor (to the myoepithelium of sweat glands) in type. They are lightly or non-myelinated.

The nerve fibres lie in bundles called funiculi. The entire nerve is invested in a sheath of loose connective tissue (epineurium) which separates the funiculi in addition. Each funiculus is surrounded by connective tissue cells known as perineurium. Within the funiculi, loose connective tissue (endoneurium) surrounds the nerve fibres.

Ganglia

The ganglia of conduction can be distinguished histologically from the ganglia of synapse. Ganglia of conduction are characterised as follows:

The nerve cells are pseudo-unipolar.

Many satellites surround the cell body.

The majority of the nerve fibres are heavily myelinated.

The cell bodies lie in clumps separated by bundles of nerve fibres.

Ganglia of synapse have the following histological features:

The nerve cells are multipolar.

Satellites are few.

The nerve fibres are non-myelinated for the most part.

The cell bodies are distributed randomly in the ganglion.

Neuroglia

The neuroglial cells are of four types:

Oligodendrocytes. These are the satellites of the cyton and the supporting cells of the axon of the neurones of the central nervous system.

Microglia. These are the scavenger cells of the central nervous system. They are of small size with many branched spiny protoplasmic processes.

Astrocytes. These cells have long cytoplasmic processes which may be fine or coarse and which determine whether the cell is classified as being fibrous or protoplasmic in type. The processes terminate in expansions on blood vessel walls and it is concluded that these cells transfer nutrients to the nerve cells in their vicinity, and form a blood-brain barrier.

Ependyma. This lines the ventricular system of the central nervous system, and is arranged in such manner as to resemble simple columnar epithelium but the ependymal cells send long branching processes from their basal regions into the underlying nervous tissue.

---

84 *Peripheral nervous system, TS mixed peripheral nerve (H & E)* The nerve fibres are gathered into a number of funiculi separated by loose connective tissue (epineurium) and surrounded by concentric connective tissue cells (perineurium).

85 *Peripheral nervous system, TS mixed peripheral nerve (Osmic acid)* The myelin sheaths are stained black by this method.

86 *Peripheral nervous system, TS mixed peripheral nerve (H & E)* A high power view of a single funiculus from **84**. The perineurium is at the top. The funiculus is composed of many medullated and some non-medullated fibres lying in loose connective tissue (endoneurium).

87 *Peripheral nervous system, TS mixed peripheral nerve (Osmic acid)* The axons appear as a clear halo surrounded by a dark ring of stained myelin.

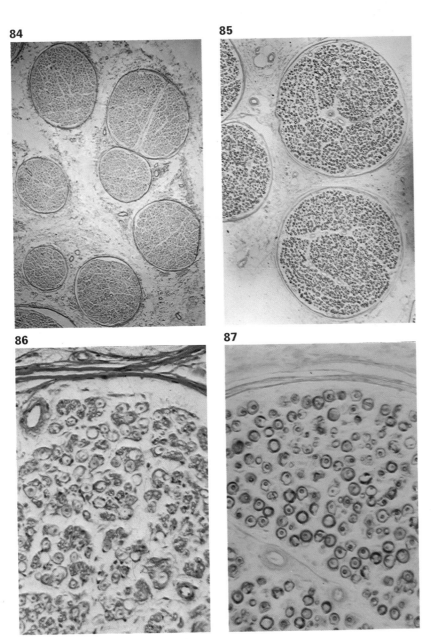

84

85

86

87

57

88 *Peripheral nervous system, LS mixed peripheral nerve (H & E)* Three funiculi are sectioned. Each is invested by (deep pink) concentric connective tissue cells (perineurium). The funiculi are separated by loose connective tissue (epineurium).

89 *Peripheral nervous system, mixed peripheral nerve, perineurium (Silver)* The connective tissue cells of the perineurium are outlined, and resemble endothelial cells.

90 *Peripheral nervous system, LS mixed peripheral nerve (H & E)* A high power view of **88** showing portions of two funiculi and their perineurium, with epineurium between. The fibres have a foamy appearance due to dissolution of the myelin. Schwann and fibroblast nuclei are present in the funiculus. A node of Ranvier lies in the funiculus on the left, just left of centre (*arrow*).

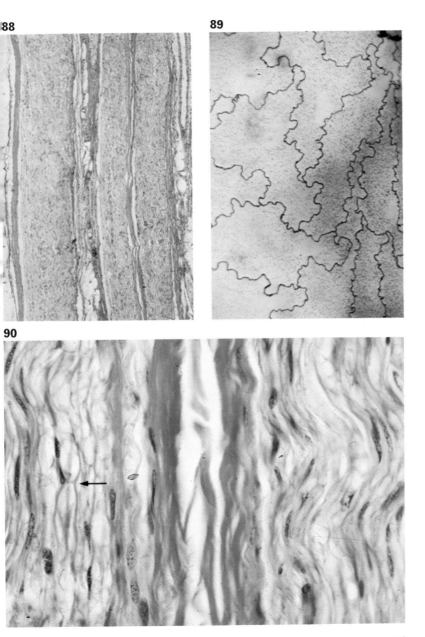

Dorsal root ganglion

91 *Peripheral nervous system, ganglion of conduction (H & E)* In this low power view of a dorsal root ganglion the clumps of nerve cells appear as dark areas and the nerve fibres as pale areas.

92 *Peripheral nervous system, ganglion of conduction (H & E)* Higher power view of **91** to show the nerve cell, and nerve fibre clumps.

93 *Peripheral nervous system, ganglion of synapse (H & E)* Under low power, no evidence of clumping of cells or fibres can be discerned in this autonomic ganglion.

Sympathetic ganglion

94 *Peripheral nervous system, ganglion of synapse (H & E)* Higher power view of **93**. The nerve cells and fibres are randomly distributed.

95 *Peripheral nervous system, ganglion of conduction (Osmic acid)* In this low power view the segregation of cells from fibres is again manifest. Dorsal root ganglion.

96 *Peripheral nervous system, ganglion of conduction (Osmic acid)* High power of **95** to show that the nerve fibres are heavily medullated since myelin stains black with osmic acid.

91

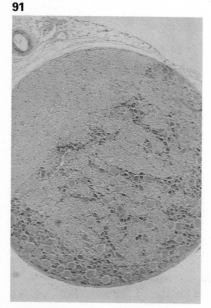

92

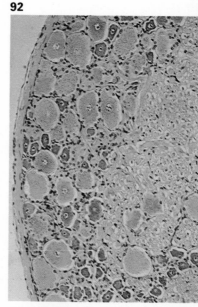

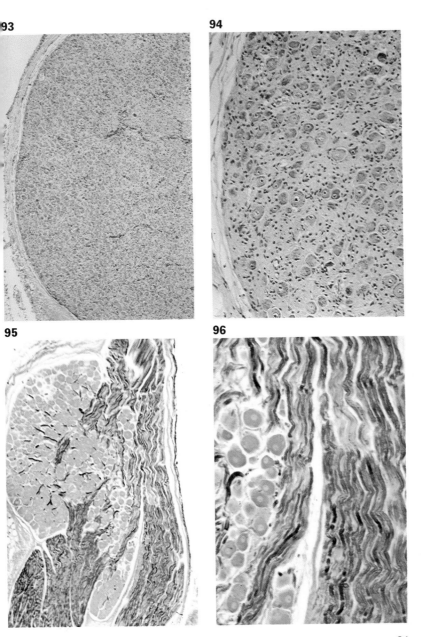

93

94

95

96

61

97 *Peripheral nervous system, ganglion of synapse (Silver)* The plexus of Auerbach in the small gut silhouetted against a background of smooth muscle cut longitudinally.

98 *Peripheral nervous system, ganglion of synapse (Silver)* High power of figure **97** to show multipolar cells lying at random in a network of fine fibres. The nuclei belong to satellite, Schwann and fibroblast cells.

99 *Peripheral nervous system, ganglion of conduction (H & E)* At high power the nerve cells are seen to have many satellite cells, and the nerve fibres to be heavily myelinated. Dorsal root ganglion.

100 *Peripheral nervous system, ganglion of synapse (H & E)* Satellites are few in number and the nerve fibres are mostly non-myelinated. Autonomic ganglion.

97

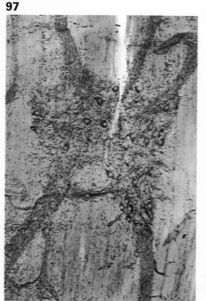

98

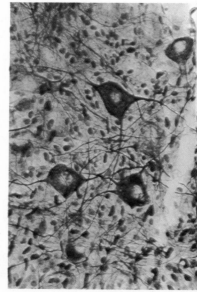

99

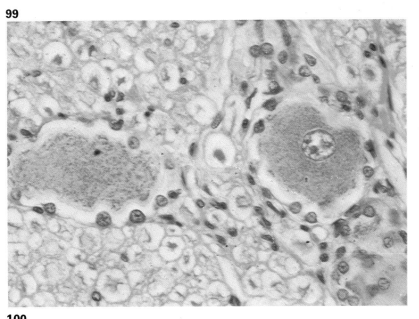

100

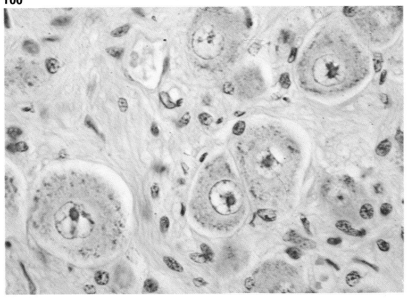

101 *Central nervous system, TS of spinal cord (Silver)* The grey matter is x-shaped, centrally located and stains dark yellow. The central canal lies in the middle of the grey matter. The white matter is almost colourless.

102 *Central nervous system, spinal cord (Silver)* High power field from **101** showing grey matter (*left*) and white matter (*right*). The grey matter has multipolar nerve cells and their processes, and neuroglial cells. The white matter is composed of medullated and non-medullated nerve fibres and neuroglial cells.

103 *Central nervous system, grey matter of spinal cord (Silver)* The multipolar nerve cells are of irregular size and shape and have a single circular nucleus.

104 *Central nervous system, grey matter of spinal cord (H & E)* The nerve cell cytoplasm is packed with masses of basophilic material (Nissl substance) except at one point (axon hillock). The neuroglial cell nuclei are dense and small by comparison with the large pale nuclei of the nerve cells.

101

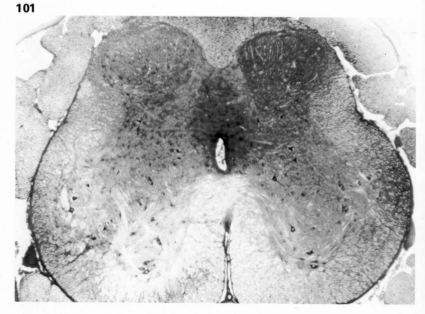

102

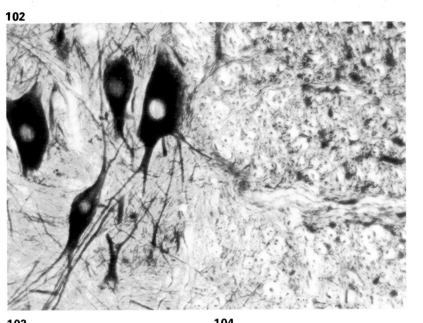

103

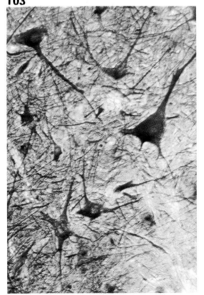

104

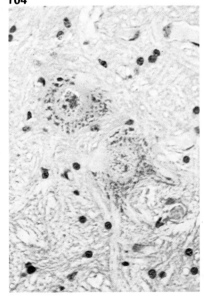

65

105 *Central nervous system, cerebellum (H & E)* The cerebellum has grey matter (cortex) superficially and white matter (medulla) deep to that. The surface is highly folded.

106 *Central nervous system, cerebellar cortex (H & E)* The molecular layer (*right*) Purkinje cell layer (*arrows*) and granular layer (*bottom left*) can be seen.

107 *Central nervous system, cerebellum (Silver)* The medulla (*bottom left*) stains dark brown. The three layers of the cortex can be seen.

108 *Central nervous system, cerebellum (Silver)* High power of cerebellar cortex. The granular layer (*bottom*) is separated from the molecular layer (*top*) by the Purkinje cells (two of which are seen) and whose dendrites ramify in the molecular layer.

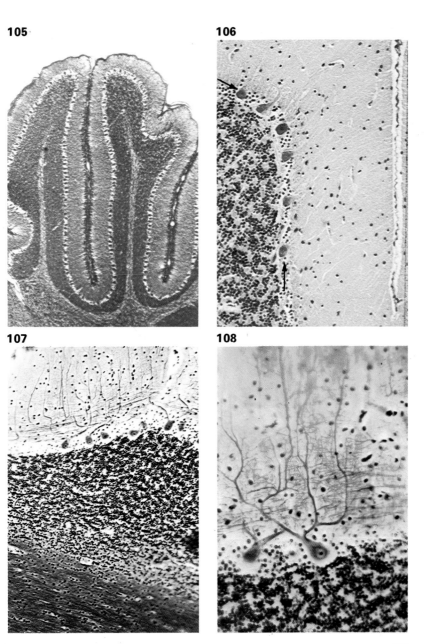

67

109 *Central nervous system, cerebral cortex (H & E)* This shows homo-typical cortex (from visual area) in which all six layers can be distinguished. Homotypical cortex occurs everywhere but in the motor and sensory areas.

110 *Central nervous system, cerebral cortex (Lithium haematoxylin)* Homotypical cortex from the visual area. Layers four and six (outer and inner bands of Baillarger) can be seen as dark bands running from left to right.

111 *Central nervous system, cerebral cortex (H & E)* In heterotypical cortex the six layers cannot be distinguished. Granular cortex of post-central gyrus (sensory area).

112 *Central nervous system, cerebral cortex (Lithium haematoxylin)* As **111**. The myelin sheaths are stained. The bundles of nerve fibres entering the white matter can be seen at the bottom of the field.

113 *Central nervous system, cerebral cortex (Silver)* Heterotypical cortex in which the nerve cell processes have been impregnated with silver.

114 *Central nervous system, neuroglia (Golgi method)* Several fibrous astrocytes can be seen.

109

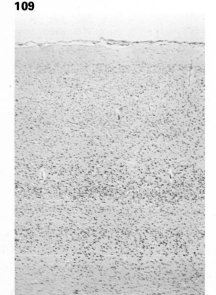

110

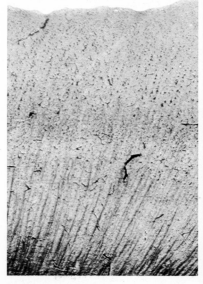

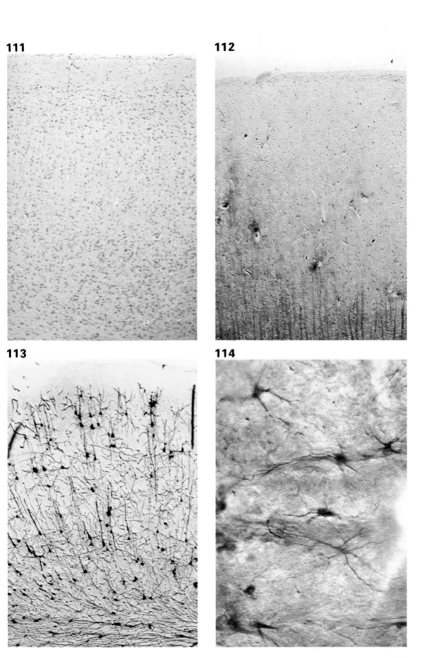

111

112

113

114

69

115 *Central nervous system, neuroglia (Golgi method)* Many protoplasmic astrocytes can be made out.

116 *Central nervous system, neuroglia (H & E)* Part of the choroid plexus to show ependymal cells.

115

116

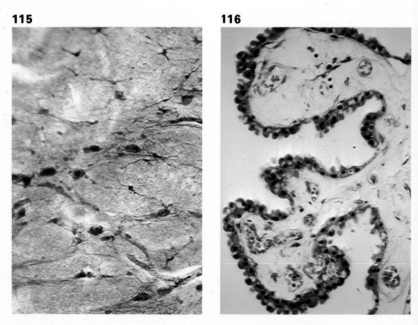

The Circulatory System

The circulatory system consists of the heart, arteries, veins, capillaries, sinusoids, and lymphatic vessels of the body. Arteries, veins and capillaries and some sinusoids (in liver, spleen and marrow) contain blood whereas lymphatic vessels and the sinuses of lymph nodes contain a clear fluid —lymph—derived from extra-cellular fluid. All blood vessels except sinusoids are lined by endothelium.

THE CAPILLARIES AND SINUSOIDS

These are near relatives but differ in some fundamental respects. They resemble one another in that they are of fine calibre, are thin-walled and permit considerable exchange of metabolites across or through their walls. They differ in the respect that capillaries have parallel continuous walls lined by endothelium whereas sinusoids have undulating discontinuous walls lined by phagocytic cells called fixed macrophages or reticulo-endothelial cells.

The electron microscopists describe capillaries as being of two types, non-fenestrated, and fenestrated. In the latter type ultra-microscopic endothelial narrowings bridged by extremely fine diaphragms are seen. These are far removed from the gaps of up to 0.5μ which occur between adjacent sinusoidal macrophages.

THE ARTERIES AND VEINS

All arteries, arterioles and veins have walls consisting of three tunics, the middle one of which (tunica media) imparts to each vessel (except in the case of the very large veins) that property which enables it to perform its particular role in the circulatory process. The inner tunic is the tunica intima and the outer, the tunica adventitia. Each tunic is composed of the same elements in both arteries and veins, but their proportions vary. The three tunics cannot be distinguished in venules.

The tunica intima
This comprises the inner endothelial lining resting on a layer of areolar tissue. The endothelial cell nuclei bulge conspicuously into the lumen of the vessel and appear circular in outline in vessels cut in transverse section and oval in vessels sectioned longitudinally. The areolar connective tissue varies in amount, being considerable in large vessels so that the tunica intima is easily recognisable, and reduced to a film in small vessels so that the tunic is difficult to distinguish.

The tunica media
This is the most substantial tunic in all blood vessels except the very large veins. It is composed of circularly-arranged smooth muscle interspersed with elastic

tissue in the form of circularly-disposed fibres, or as concentric sheets (lamellae) or both. The proportions of the muscular and elastic elements vary widely from vessel to vessel. Arteries can be distinguished from veins because they invariably possess a lamella of elastic tissue immediately deep to the tunica intima and called the internal elastic lamina. This structure is not found in any vein. Larger arteries also possess a similar lamina of elastic tissue at the outer edge of the tunica media where it abuts on the tunica adventitia: this is called the external elastic lamina and it too is never seen in veins.

The tunica adventitia

This tunic is composed of longitudinally-arranged collagen and elastic fibres and cells of the fibroblast type. Large veins and certain muscular arteries (splenic, renal and superior mesenteric) additionally possess bundles of longitudinally-disposed smooth muscle fibres in the tunica adventitia. Blood vessels known as vasa vasorum are found in this tunic.

Nutrition of arteries and veins

This is accomplished by diffusion. The inner half of the wall of a vessel is nourished from the lumen and the outer half from the vasa vasorum. Diffusion into vessels in the contracted stage will be poor, with the result that degenerative changes in blood vessel walls are commonplace.

Arteries

Arteries are of two types: elastic and muscular. The smallest vessels of the arterial tree are called arterioles. Blood is pumped through arteries by contraction of the ventricles (i.e. during systole) and during diastole by the recoil of the large juxta-cardiac arteries which have considerable amounts of elastic tissue in their wall. These elastic arteries comprise the aorta and the brachiocephalic, common carotid, subclavian, pulmonary, common iliac and vertebral arteries. Muscular arteries are sometimes called arteries of distribution as their tunica media is composed largely of smooth muscle, the variations in tone of which regulate the flow of blood to the parts supplied by the vessel. All the named arteries in the body except those listed above under elastic arteries are of this type. The transition from elastic to muscular artery is gradual so that vessels possessing characteristics intermediate between the two types may be seen. As to the arterioles, they are unnamed and characterised by the fact that the thickness of their wall is greater than the diameter of their lumen. This equips them well for their task of stepping-down the arterial blood pressure so that the capillaries receive blood at a pressure which will not rupture their wall.

Veins

Veins are more numerous than arteries and are of greater calibre than their accompanying artery because the rate of blood flow in veins is much slower than in arteries. The largest veins pursue courses independent from, and usually have names different from, those of the corresponding elastic arteries. The medium sized veins are named according to their accompanying artery. The smallest veins, or venules, run with the arterioles but are not named. The veins of the limbs have one-way valves at intervals along their length. When muscular activity occurs in the limb the vein is compressed against the deep fascia and blood is forced past the valves: to facilitate the process the wall of the vein is composed largely of collagen and is relatively indistensible. The blood is moved along the veins of the trunk by the sucking effect generated during expiration: the veins of the thorax and abdomen are therefore devoid of valves. The veins of the head and neck rarely possess valves.

Venous valves
These are usually bicuspid, sometimes tricuspid. Distal to the valve is a slight dilatation of the vein. The cusps are extensions of the tunica intima—i.e. they have a core of areolar tissue and are covered by endothelium.

Lymph vessels
These commence as blindly-ending capillaries which unite to form vessels of progressively increasing size which discharge finally into the venous system. The capillaries are tubes of mere endothelium. The larger lymph vessels have walls very similar to small veins—i.e. with a small amount of circular smooth muscle. The larger lymph vessels possess bicuspid valves. The fluid in the lumen is clear, being derived by transudation of extra-cellular fluid.

Arteriovenous anastomoses
These represent connections between arterioles and venules and are of two types:
Glomus or Hoyer-Sucquet anastomoses. These are found in the lips, nose, nail bed, fingers and toes. There is a connecting vessel between the arteriole and venule which is either very tortuous or may divide into up to six branches: either way the anastomosis is arranged in a spherical mass or glomus. The smooth muscle of the tunica media of the arteriolar end of the connecting vessel is greatly modified in that the fibres branch and form a syncytium. The venous end of the connecting vessel consists of endothelium resting on a thin fibro-elastic membrane.
Direct type. Arteriovenous anastomoses of this nature are found in the vessels of the alimentary canal where the intermittent metabolic activity seems to render their presence necessary. The arteriole opens directly into the venule, there being no interconnecting vessels.

THE HEART

The wall of the heart is composed of three layers: an inner endocardium, a middle myocardium and an outer epicardium which correspond roughly to the three tunics of blood vessels.

The endocardium
This is composed of the endothelial lining of the heart chamber resting on areolar tissue. The conducting tissue of the heart lies in the areolar tissue of the endocardium.

The myocardium
This is composed of cardiac muscle and varies in its degree of development from chamber to chamber.

The epicardium
This layer is thicker than the endocardium. It consists of the endothelium of the visceral pericardial layer resting on areolar tissue. Deep to this is dense connective tissue in the case of the atria and adipose tissue in the instance of the ventricles. The coronary arteries lie embedded in this adipose tissue.

The heart valves
These lie either at the commencement of the aorta and pulmonary artery (semilunar valves) or between the atria and ventricles (atrioventricular valves). The valves consist of a core of loose connective tissue sandwiched between the dense connective tissue of the upper and lower surfaces of the valve. The surface of the valve is covered by endothelium. The valves are largely avascular. The atrioventricular valves have the chordae tendineae attached to their ventricular aspect.

The carotid sinus
At or near its bifurcation the common carotid artery displays intimal thinning and adventitial thickening: the adventitia here contains large numbers of

continued

117 *Elastic artery (H & E)* The tunica intima is at the top (A). The tunica media (B) forms the major part of the wall of the vessel. The tunica adventitia (C) contains the vasa vasorum (D).

118 *Elastic artery (Van Gieson)* Muscle is stained yellow by this method. The tunica media is seen to possess a large complement of smooth muscle, the nuclei of which stand out.

119 *Elastic artery (Weigert's elastic)* The elastic lamellae of the tunica media are well demonstrated in this preparation.

120 *Elastic artery (Verhoeff's elastic)* The elastic lamellae of the tunica media again are well displayed.

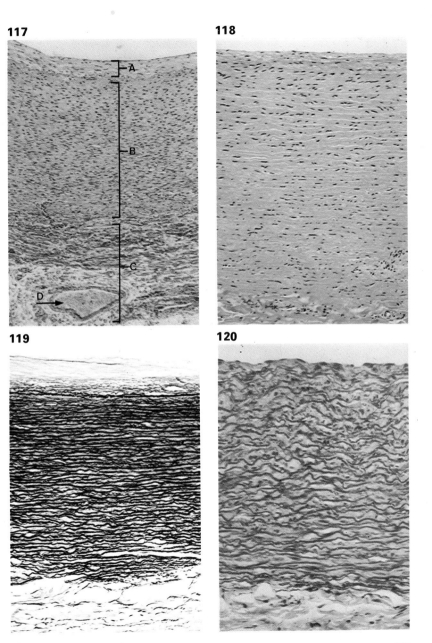

75

sensory (pressure) nerve-endings derived from the glossopharyngeal nerve.

The carotid body

This is a spherical pea-sized organ found in the angle of bifurcation of the common carotid artery. It is composed of clumps of connective tissue cells with epithelial-like appearance and the mass is richly innervated by the glossopharyngeal nerve. It responds to alterations in the chemical composition of the blood. Two bodies (aortic) of similar structure are found near the origin of the subclavian arteries.

---

121 *Muscular artery (H & E)* The tunica intima (A) is less extensive than in arteries of the elastic type. The tunica media (B) is composed mainly of smooth muscle, the nuclei of which can be seen. The tunica adventitia (C) is mainly collagenous.

122 *Muscular artery (Van Gieson)* The tunica intima (A) is stained pink and is separated from the tunica media by the internal elastic lamina (B). The tunica media (C) stains yellow, and some elastic fibres lie in its outer part. The collagenous adventitia (D) stains red.

123 *Muscular artery (H & OGE)* The stain employed stains the elastic tissue bright pink. The internal elastic lamina is seen at A and the elastic fibres of the tunica adventitia at B.

124 *Muscular artery (Weigert's elastic)* Elastic tissue is here stained black. The internal elastic lamina (A) is well delineated. The tunica adventitia has a high content of elastic fibres.

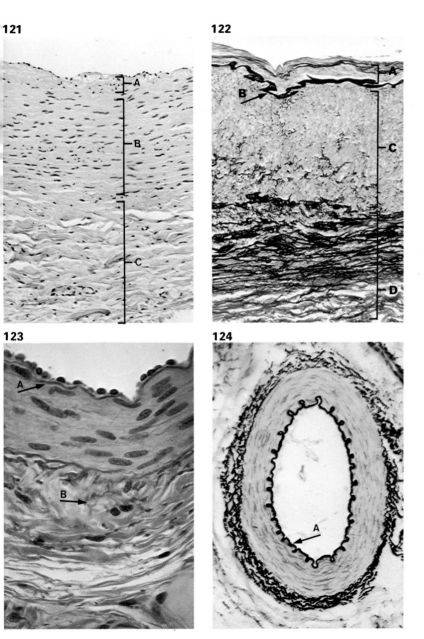

121

122

123

124

125 *LS arteriole (H & E)* The elongated nuclei of the lining endothelial cells are seen at A. The nuclei of the smooth muscle cells of the tunica media appear at B.

126 *TS arterioles (H & E)* Profiles of two arterioles are seen. The endothelial nuclei (A) are circular when cut transversely. The nuclei of the smooth muscle cells (B) extend for some distance around the circumference of the vessel.

127 *TS capillaries (H & E)* In this field are several capillaries. The dark nuclei of their endothelial lining cells can be seen (*arrows*).

128 *LS capillaries (Silver)* On the left is a skeletal muscle fibre, and on the right is a bundle of collagen. Between these lie capillaries filled with erythrocytes.

125

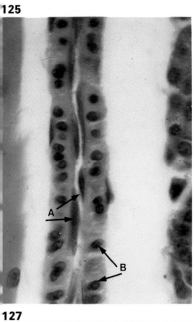

126

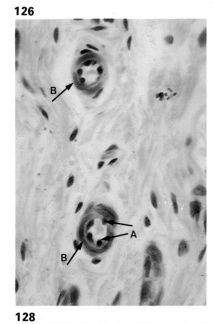

127

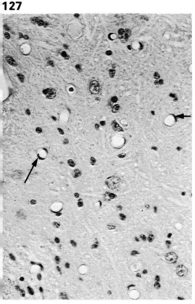

128

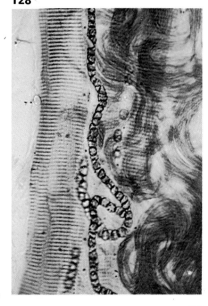

129 *Large vein (H & E)* The tunica intima (A) is composed of loose connective tissue. The tunica media (B) has some circular smooth muscle. The tunica adventitia (C) possesses longitudinal smooth muscle (D).

130 *Medium vein and muscular artery (H & E)* The vein (*top*) has a thinner wall than its accompanying artery (*bottom*). A valve is present in the vein.

131 *Medium vein (Elastic stain)* High power of the vein in **130**. The endothelial nuclei (A) are the most obvious feature of the tunica intima. The tunica media (B) contains smooth muscle (C) and elastic fibres (D). The tunica adventitia (E) contains collagen and elastic fibres.

132 *Venous valve (H & E)* In this small vein a valve with two cusps is seen. The valve is composed of connective tissue covered by endothelium.

133 *Arteriovenous anastomosis (H & OGE)* Arteriovenous anastomoses of the direct type, as here, are uncommon in man.

129

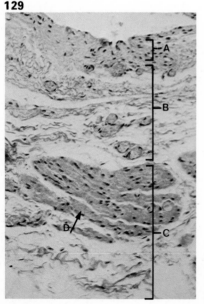

130

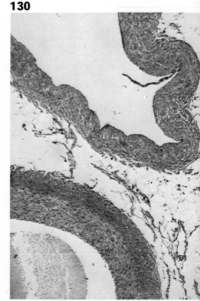

131

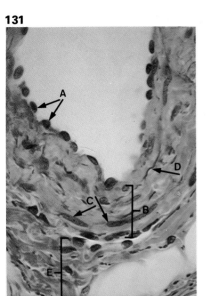

132

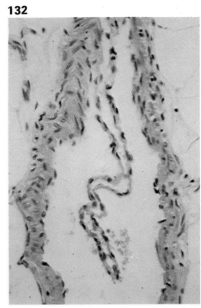

133

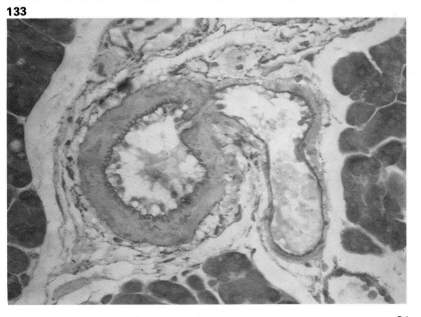

134 *Arteriovenous anastomosis (Iron haematoxylin)* An arteriovenous anastomosis of the glomus type is shown. The connecting vessels between artery and vein have modified walls (*see page 73*). The arterial end of the connecting vessel is seen at A and the venous end at B.

135 *Carotid sinus (Van Gieson)* The unmodified common carotid artery (typical elastic) lies on the left. On the right is the commencement of the carotid sinus in which the elastic lamellae are absent from the tunica media except in its outer portion.

136 *Carotid body (H & E)* At the top is the internal carotid artery. The carotid body occupies the lower half of the field. Its artery of supply lies on its right.

137 *Carotid body (H & E)* A high power of **136** to show the connective tissue cells of the carotid body (glomus cells). They are arranged in a manner reminiscent of epithelium.

134

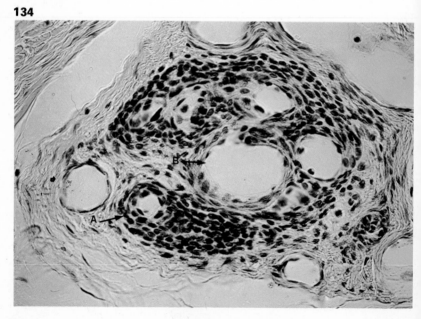

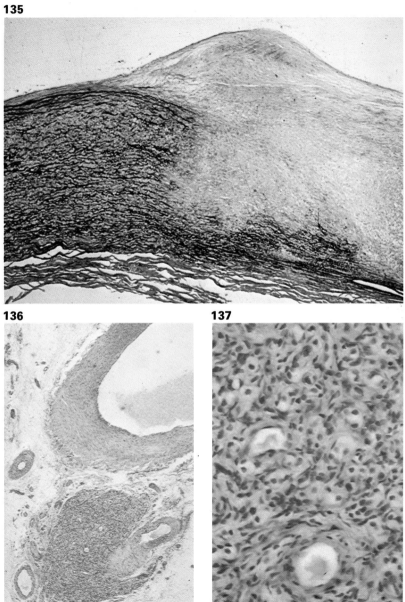

135

136

137

83

138 *Heart, epicardium (H & E)* The epicardium comprises the endothelium of the visceral layer of the pericardium (A) resting on areolar tissue (B) in which lie the coronary blood vessels (C). The myocardium is seen at D.

139 *Heart, endocardium (Azan)* The endocardium is composed of the endothelial lining of the chambers of the heart (A) resting on loose connective tissue (B). Myocardium is present at C.

140 *Heart, atrioventricular node (H & E)* The atrioventricular and sino-atrial nodes comprise tangled Purkinje fibres (A) with connective tissue between (B

141 *Heart, valves (H & E)* The semilunar valves (A) lie at the root of the great vessels which are arteries of the elastic type (B). The atrioventricular valves (C) lie between the atrium (D) and the ventricle (E). A coronary artery lies at F.

142 *Heart, semilunar valve (H & E)* The valve is composed of loose connective tissue (A) with dense connective tissue on its lower surface (B) and especially its upper surface (C).

143 *Heart, semilunar valve (H & E)* High power of **142**. The endothelial covering of the valve can be seen (A).

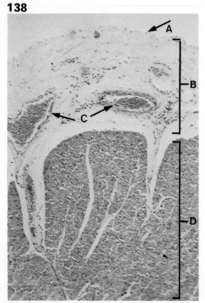

138

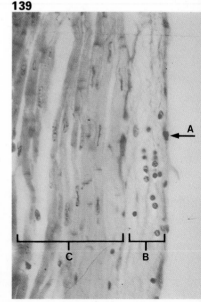

139

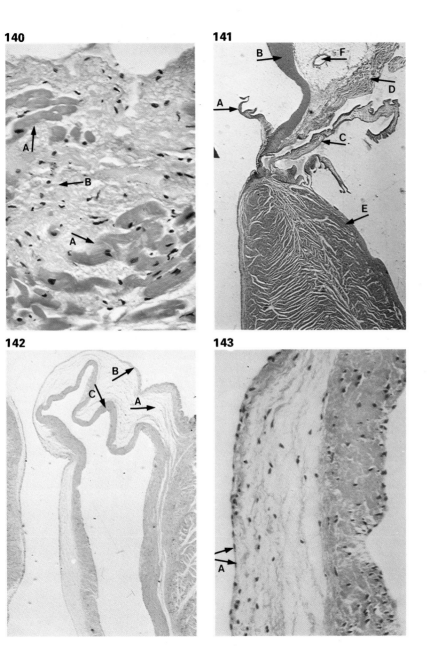

144 *Heart, atrioventricular valve (Azan)* The valve is composed of loose connective tissue covered by endothelium. Collagen is stained blue. The valve has a series of tendons (chordae tendineae) attached to its ventricular surface (A).

145 *Heart, atrioventricular valve (Azan)* High power of **144** to show the strip of dense connective tissue on the underside of the valve (A).

144

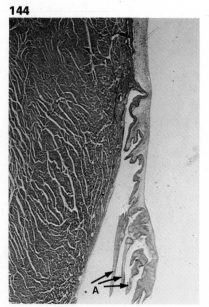

145

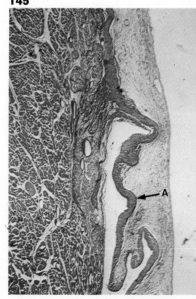

The Lymphomyeloid Complex

THE BLOOD

Blood is a loose connective tissue in which the intercellular substance is fluid, and is called plasma. Plasma is homogeneous under the microscope and constitutes 55% of the total blood volume of 6 litres. It contains minute fat droplets (known as chylomicrons) globulins and albumins. When blood is exposed to air, one of the globulins known as fibrinogen becomes precipitated and eventually converted to threads of fibrin, leaving behind the serum, a clear straw-coloured fluid.

The cells of the blood are of two types, red blood corpuscles or erythrocytes and white blood corpuscles or leucocytes. In addition one encounters the blood platelets, which are particles of cytoplasm derived from bone marrow giant cells.

The erythrocytes

These number 10^6 per mm³. Each is a biconcave disc of 7.5µ in diameter, and contains the pigment haemoglobin. A single erythrocyte is of pale yellow colour: it is only when they are in the mass that they appear red. The red cells are extremely elastic and flexible, properties which they require to enable them to pass along capillaries whose diameter is often less than theirs. They are anucleate.

The leucocytes

The white cells are not demonstrated well by H & E. Special stains (e.g. Wright's) based on eosin and methylene blue are needed to display them. The leucocytes can be divided into two subclasses according to whether they possess cytoplasmic granules or not. There are between 4,000 and 10,000 white cells in each cubic millimetre of blood. All the white cells seem to be able to enter and leave the blood stream by crossing the wall of a capillary.

Agranular leucocytes These are of two types:
Lymphocytes. Small (6–8µ) and medium (8–10µ) lymphocytes are found in the blood and between them account for 20–30% of the total leucocyte count. They have a single spherical nucleus which almost fills the cell: the nuclear chromatin is located characteristically around the periphery of the nucleus. The cytoplasm is a mere rim in small lymphocytes and rather more abundant in medium lymphocytes. In both it is agranular.
Monocytes. These cells belong to the macrophage system of the body, and therefore are actively phagocytic. When they leave the blood stream to enter the tissues they are known as histiocytes or wandering cells. They are the largest of the leucocytes, being of some 15–20µ in diameter. They number some 2–8% of the total leucocyte population. There is a single reniform nucleus and abundant pale and rather featureless cytoplasm.

Granular leucocytes The granular leucocytes are of three types and all possess nuclei which are subdivided into at least two distinct lobes—i.e. they are polymorphonuclear.

Neutrophil polymorphs. These are the most numerous of the leucocytes, 60–70% of which are of this type. The cell is 10–12μ in diameter and the nucleus becomes progressively more lobed with age. As many as five lobes may be seen. The cells are phagocytic and are sometimes called microphages. They have a pale cytoplasm containing fine brownish granules. They are found in large numbers in any acute inflammatory process and can phagocytose bacteria. Neutrophils are the chief constituent of pus.

Eosinophil polymorphs. These are of the same order of size as the neutrophils and the basophils (i.e. 10–12μ) but form only 2% of the total white cell population. They have a bilobed nucleus and the cytoplasm is crammed with large eosinophilic granules. The function of these cells is unknown. They are found in increased numbers in the blood of persons suffering from allergic states such as asthma and hay fever.

Basophil polymorphs. These are the least common of all the cells of the blood, accounting for less than $\frac{1}{2}$% of the total white count. . The cells have a bilobed nucleus and many large basophilic granules lie in the cytoplasm. Some authorities think they are mast cells, but most would not agree. Their function is unknown.

The blood platelets

These are cytoplasmic particles of some 2–3u in diameter derived from the cytoplasm of the bone marrow giant cells. There are up to 800,000 platelets per cubic millimetre of blood. They are important in plugging gaps in the vascular tree, which they do because they appear to be adhesive and to have surface barbs which foul on the precipitated fibrin. They also participate in the formation of thromboplastin in the process of blood clotting.

THE BONE MARROW

Bone marrow may be yellow or red in type. Yellow bone marrow is composed of adipose tissue and red bone marrow of adipose tissue and haematopoietic tissue in admixture. Blood sinusoids lined by fixed macrophages (reticulo-endothelial cells) are found in red bone marrow.

The haemopoietic tissue is responsible for the production of the blood cells of the myeloid (i.e. red cells and granular leucocytes) lymphoid and monocyte series, as well as the platelets of the blood. All develop in all probability from a common ancestor, the bone marrow stem cell or haemocytoblast.

Erythrocytes

The stem cell gives rise via a postulated intermediary, the pro-erythroblast, to normoblasts of early, intermediate and late type. The early normoblast (or basophil erythroblast) has a spherical nucleus with chromatin distributed in draught-board fashion and a deeply basophilic cytoplasm: with the E.M. the cytoplasm is seen to be rich in rough-surfaced endoplasmic reticulum. The early normoblast divides to give rise to the intermediate normoblast (or polychromatophil erythroblast) which has a similar nucleus but the cytoplasm now contains a quantity of haemoglobin whose eosinophilia neutralises the basophilia so that the cytoplasm is of a dirty grey colour. The intermediate normoblast divides to give rise to the late normoblast which looks like a large nucleated erythrocyte and which is incapable of mitosis. It extrudes its nucleus to become a reticulocyte. By supra-vital staining with a dye such as cresyl violet, a network, the residue of the rough E.R., can be demonstrated in the cytoplasm of these cells, which form 1% of the circulating erythrocytes. Reticulocytes become erythrocytes on losing this reticulum.

Granular leucocytes

These develop from haemocytoblasts via another postulated intermediary, the myeloblast. This gives rise to promyelocytes which have a spherical nucleus and a few cytoplasmic granules which in any given cell may be neutrophil or eosinophil or basophil in nature. The promyelocytes divide to give rise to myelocytes which have a kidney-shaped nucleus and which have a greater quantity of granules of the specific type. The myelocytes in turn divide to give rise to metamyelocytes which have a bilobed nucleus and an even greater concentration of specific granules. They are incapable of division. They transform into adult polymorphs of the specific type, according to their granule content.

Monocytes

These develop from haemocytoblasts via a postulated intermediary, the monoblast. They enter the blood stream and reach the vascularised tissues where they emerge to become free macrophages (histiocytes) or fixed macrophages (reticulo-endothelial cells) of lymph nodes, spleen, liver and bone marrow.

Lymphocytes
The origin of these cells is described below under thymus.

The blood platelets
The haemocytoblast gives rise to bone marrow giant cells which may be uni-nucleate (megakaryocytes) or multinucleate (polykaryocytes) and which form the platelets of the blood by liberating small portions of their cytoplasm into the marrow sinusoids.

THE THYMUS

The thymus is a primary lymphoid organ, and so exhibits the following characteristics:

It contains epithelial cells which elaborate a hormone necessary for the proper development of the thymic lymphocytes.

It exhibits lymphopoiesis which is of greater intensity than that seen in secondary lymphoid organs and which is independent of antigenic stimulation.

It does not possess lymph nodules or plasma cells.

It receives lymphoid stem cells (lymphoblasts) from the bone marrow early in foetal life. Lymphocytes make their appearance in the foetal thymus before doing so in the foetal secondary lymphoid organs.

Thymic resection before or at birth results in severe immunological crippling which can be reversed only by inoculating lymphoid stem cells.

The thymus is covered by a capsule of connective tissue which dips into the organ dividing it into a large number of lobules. The gland has an outer cortex and an inner medulla, and in both are found cells of epithelial, lymphoid and macrophage types.

The cortex The cortex is darker than the medulla because of its greater concentration of lymphoid cells. These cells exhibit a gradient of both size and mitotic activity from without inwards. The large, actively dividing lymphoblasts are nearest the surface. These divide to give rise to large lymphocytes which multiply in turn to give rise to medium lymphocytes. Their progeny, the small lymphocytes, occupy the deepest part of the cortex. Epithelial cells in a reticular network occupy the interstices between the lymphoid cells. Occasional free macrophages also occur.

The medulla The medulla is composed of small lymphocytes and a network of stellate epithelial cells. Some free macrophages are again present. Peculiar to the medulla are epithelial ovoids of some 20/50 microns in diameter and known as the corpuscles of Hassall. They are composed of concentrically arranged epithelial cells which are commonly hyalinised and degenerate. Their peripheral cells extend outwards to join the medullary epithelial cell network. The function of the corpuscles of Hassall is unknown.

The small lymphocytes of the thymic medulla enter the blood stream to form the pool of long-lived circulating lymphocytes. They emerge from the capillaries and sinusoids of lymph nodes and spleen respectively to populate the thymus-dependent areas of these organs. They are responsible for cell-mediated immune responses.

The bursa of Fabricius
This primary lymphoid organ is present only in birds. It has a histological appearance almost identical to that of the thymus. The lymphocytes it produces populate the bursa-dependent areas of the secondary lymphoid organs and so give rise to the lymph nodules and the plasma cells, which are responsible for serum-mediated immune responses. The equivalent organ in mammals is as yet in dispute, but the tonsils, appendix, foetal liver and Peyer's patches could meet the requirements in that they all have intimate epithelio-lymphocytic arrangements.

THE LYMPH NODES AND SPLEEN

These are secondary lymphoid organs and so exhibit the following characteristics:

They do not possess epithelial cells.

Lymphopoiesis is less intense than in the primary lymphoid organs and takes place only after stimulation by antigen.

Lymph nodules and plasma cells are present.

They receive lymphocytes from the primary lymphoid organs late in foetal life.

Ablation is not associated with immunological crippling and lymphoid repopulation can be achieved by inocula lacking stem cells.

The lymph nodes

These are of the size and shape of a haricot bean. They are covered by a capsule of connective tissue which is pierced over most of its extent by ingoing (afferent) lymph vessels and at the hilum by a single outgoing (efferent) lymphatic. The capsule sends collagenous trabeculae into the superficial part of the convex aspect of the node. The framework of the organ is composed of a rich network of reticular fibres. Closely attached to these fibres are fixed macrophages (reticulo-endothelial cells). The macrophages frame the lymphatic sinuses of the node which are subdivided rather artificially into subcapsular, paratrabecular and medullary groups. The lymphoid tissue is found in superficial cortical and deeper paracortical masses. The cortical lymphoid tissue consists of the lymph nodules with their germinal centres and is the bursa-dependent part: it is responsible for serum-mediated immune responses. The paracortical lymphoid tissue consists of the diffuse lymphoid masses between, and deep to the lymph nodules. It is thymus-dependent and consists of the long-lived circulating small lymphocytes which effect cell-mediated immune responses. The lymphoid sinuses are similar in all areas. They are lined by fixed macrophages whose cytoplasmic processes ramify along the network of reticular fibres. The lumen of the sinuses contains clear lymph and many small lymphocytes.

The spleen

The spleen is covered by serosal endothelium resting on a thick fibromuscular capsule containing smooth muscle, collagen and elastic fibres. From the capsule, a network of trabeculae of similar composition passes to all parts of the spleen. The large branches of the splenic artery and vein run in the trabeculae.

Between the trabeculae is a network of reticular fibres supporting the splenic parenchyma or pulp which is subdivisible into red and white portions.

The white pulp This is the lymphoid tissue of the spleen and may occur in diffuse or nodular form. The nodules may or may not possess a germinal centre. In man the demarcating line between red and white pulp is not sharp. The splenic artery sends arteriolar branches into the pulp, and these invariably enter the white pulp initially, where they are known as central arterioles: they are rarely in the centre of the lymphoid mass, however. The lymphocytes and plasma cells of the white pulp form the adventitial coat of the vessel: the central arteriole with its cuff of lymphoid tissue forms a composite known as a Malpighian corpuscle. The arteriole gives off many capillaries for the supply of the white pulp. The arteriole finally leaves the white pulp and enters the red.

The red pulp The red pulp is composed of a meshwork of reticular fibres and reticulo-endothelial cells with blood in the interstices. The blood spaces are called splenic sinusoids. They receive their blood from the penicillus arterioles, which are the extension into the red pulp of the central arterioles of the white pulp. Each central arteriole gives rise to a number of penicilli which are straight and have three parts. The first part is the arteriole of the pulp, is the longest and has a tunica intima of smooth muscle: its adventitia is formed by the sinusoids of the red pulp. The second part or sheathed arteriole is devoid of smooth muscle and is surrounded instead by an elliptical mass of concentrically-arranged reticular fibres and reticulo-endothelial cells. The third part is the so-called arteriolar capillary, and is composed of tall endothelial cells with wide spaces between. The splenic sinusoids are drained by venous sinuses, lined by endothelium. The venous sinuses open into the trabecular veins which are endothelial channels supported by the fibromuscular tissue of the trabeculae.

146 *Blood film, small lymphocyte (Wright's)* The cell is little larger than the erythrocytes. The nucleus practically fills the cell.

147 *Blood film, medium lymphocyte (Wright's)* The cell is considerably larger than the erythrocytes and has more abundant cytoplasm than a small lymphocyte.

148 *Blood film, monocyte, platelets (Wright's)* The monocyte (*top*) is the largest cell in the blood. It has a single reniform nucleus and abundant cytoplasm devoid of any granule content. Platelets (*bottom*) are cytoplasmic particles.

149 *Blood film, basophil polymorph (Wright's)* The nucleus is bilobed but is largely obscured by very big basophil granules in the overlying cytoplasm.

150 *Blood film, neutrophil polymorph (Wright's)* The nucleus is multi-lobed. The cytoplasm contains fine granules.

151 *Blood film, eosinophil polymorph (Wright's)* The nucleus is bilobed. The cytoplasm is crammed with large eosinophil granules.

146

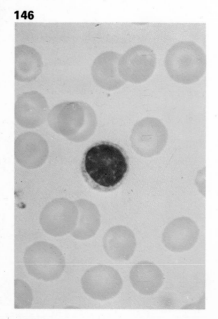

147

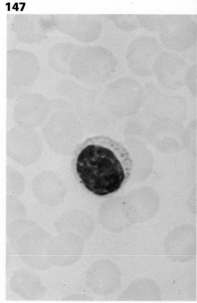

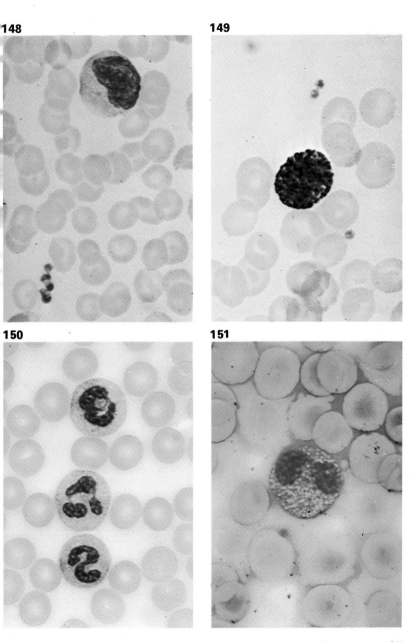

148

149

150

151

95

152 *Blood film, neutrophil and eosinophil (Wright's)* The contrast in granule size between the neutrophil (*top*) and the eosinophil (*bottom*) is apparent in this field.

153 *Blood film, polymorphonuclear leucocytes (Wright's)* The neutrophil (*top*) eosinophil (*below left*) and basophil (*below right*) can be distinguished by the size and colour of their granules.

154 *Red bone marrow section (H & E)* Red bone marrow contains fat cells with islands of haematopoietic tissue between. A bone marrow giant cell is seen (A) but the other cells are not differentiated by this stain.

155 *Red bone marrow film (Leishman)* The erythrocytes are grey, anucleate and homogeneous. The myriad red and white cell precursors constitute the nucleated cell population.

156 *Thymus (H & E)* The gland is highly lobulated and possesses an outer cortex, staining darkly (A), and an inner medulla, staining less intensely (B).

157 *Medulla of thymus (H & E)* The medulla is composed of epithelial cells (A) and lymphoid cells (B) in admixture. The corpuscles of Hassall (C) are epithelial structures exhibiting a wide range of size and morphology.

152

153

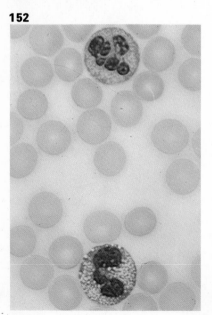
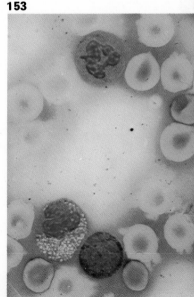

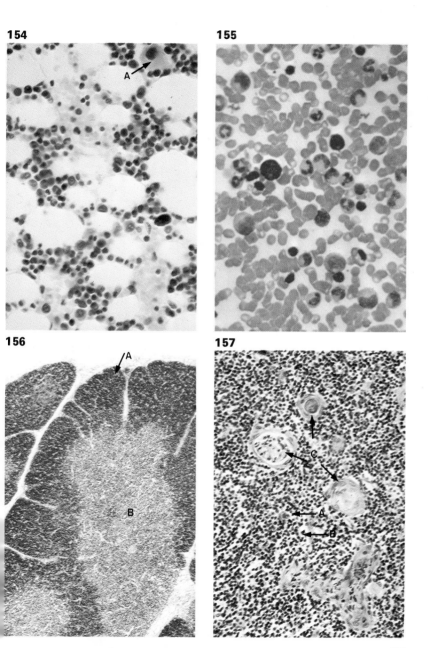

154

155

156

157

158 *Lymph node (H & E)* The node is composed of cortex (A), paracortex (B) and medulla (C).

159 *Lymph node (Azan)* As **158**.

160 *Lymph node, afferent lymphatic (H & E)* High power of **158** to show an afferent lymphatic (A) with valve (B) entering the lymph node.

161 *Lymph node, afferent lymphatic (Azan)* As **160**.

162 *Lymph node, subcapsular sinus (H & E)* The collagenous capsule (A) is separated from the cortex (B) by the subcapsular sinus (C). Fixed macrophages (reticulo-endothelial cells) bridge the sinus (D), and lymphocytes (E) lie in the sinus lumen.

158

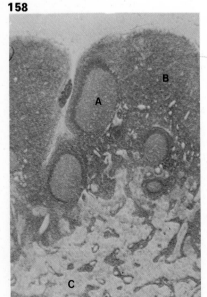

159

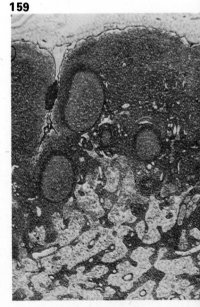

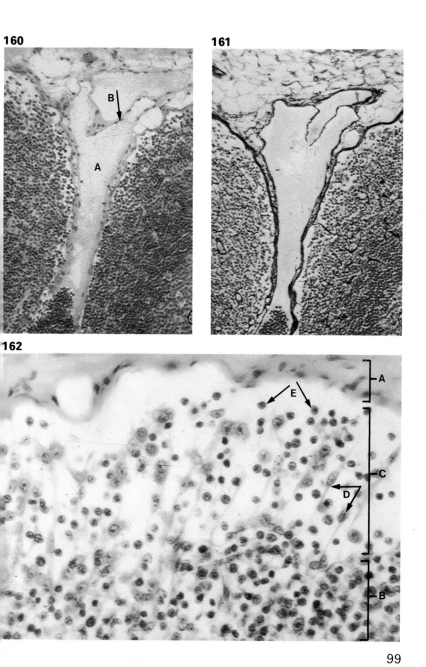

99

163 *Lymph node, subcapsular sinus (Azan)* As **162**.

164 *Lymph node, lymphatic nodule (H & E)* High power of a field from **158** showing a lymphatic nodule with germinal centre (A) and cuff of lympho-cytes (B).

165 *Lymph node, lymphatic nodule (Azan)* As **164**.

166 *Lymph node medulla (H & E)* High power view of a field from **158** showing part of a medullary cord (A) and medullary sinuses (B).

167 *Lymph node, medulla (Azan)* As **166**. The reticulo-endothelial cells (A) and reticular fibres (B) are well displayed by this stain.

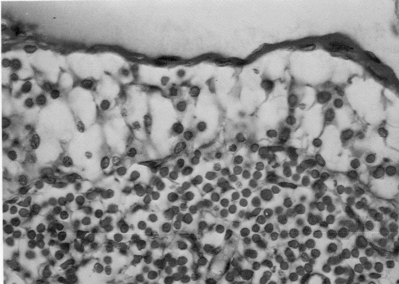

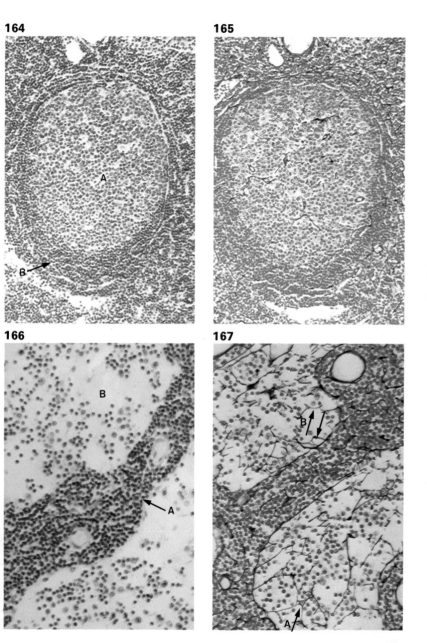

101

168 *Spleen (Van Gieson)* The capsule (A) is thicker than in lymph nodes. The red pulp (B) forms the bulk of the spleen. The white pulp (C) is the lymphoid tissue of the spleen and is distributed at random. It may take the form of nodules with germinal centres (D) or be diffuse (E).

169 *Spleen (H & E)* As **168**.

170 *Spleen, red pulp (Van Gieson)* The red pulp is composed of splenic sinusoids full of blood and lined by fixed macrophages, but it is difficult to make these features out under the light microscope.

171 *Spleen, red pulp (H & E)* The capsule (A) of the spleen is fibro-muscular. Deep to the capsule is red pulp.

172 *Spleen, white pulp (Van Gieson)* This field shows the lymphoid tissue to take the form of a lymph nodule with a germinal centre.

173 *Spleen, white pulp (H & E)* The lymphoid tissue is again in the form of a lymph nodule with a germinal centre. A tangential cut of a central arteriole is seen at A.

168

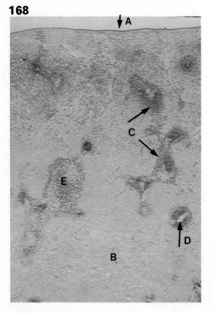

169

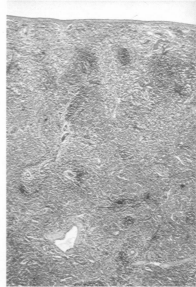

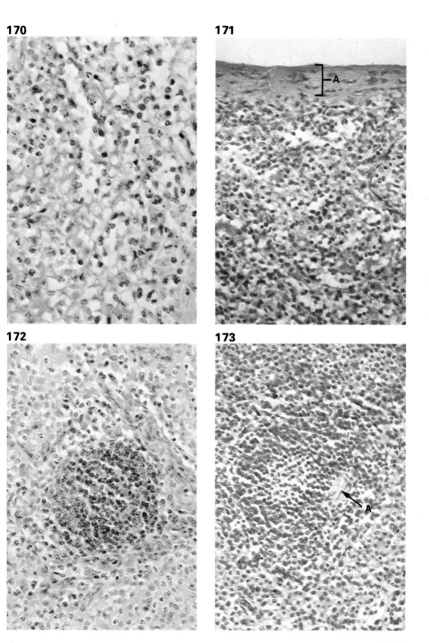

170

171

⌐A

172

173

←A

103

174 *Spleen, white pulp (Van Gieson)* The lymphoid tissue is here diffuse.

175 *Spleen, white pulp (H & E)* As **174**.

176 *Spleen, splenic artery (Van Gieson)* The splenic artery is merely an endothelial-lined space in a trabecula, the fibromuscular tissue of which acts as the vessel wall.

177 *Spleen, splenic artery (H & E)* As **176**.

178 *Spleen, sheathed arterioles (Azan)* Sheathed arterioles are poorly developed in human spleen. In this preparation of cat spleen they are prominent (A).

179 *Spleen, venous sinus (H & E)* An endothelial-lined venous sinus (A) is seen draining the red pulp (B) into the trabecular vein (C).

174   **175**

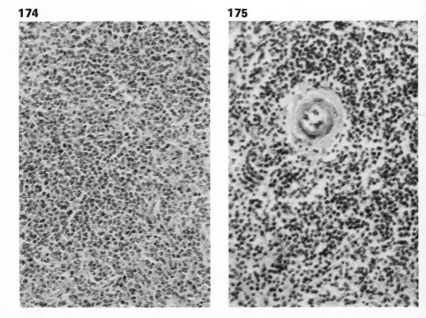

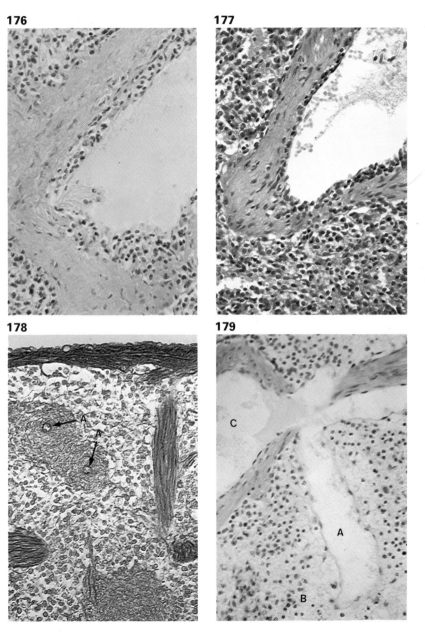

176

177

178

179

The Endocrine Glands

The endocrine tissue of the body occurs in three forms:

As discrete glands which are purely endocrine in function—the thyroid, parathyroid, adrenal and pituitary glands. These will be described in the following pages.

As endocrine portions of organs or glands which have functions additional to their endocrine one—the placenta, ovary, testis, pancreas, liver and thymus. These are described in the relevant chapters.

As isolated endocrine cells found amongst the lining epithelial cells of the alimentary canal.

The endocrine glands are (with the exception of the pars nervosa of the pituitary which is composed of white matter) composed of clusters of *epithelial* cells closely applied to fenestrated blood capillaries. The secretions of the gland are known as hormones and are discharged into the blood stream to influence the behaviour of distant (target) organs.

THE THYROID AND PARATHYROID GLANDS

The thyroid gland
This gland lies in the lower part of the front of the neck. It is enclosed in a capsule of connective tissue. The gland parenchyma comprises many spherical vesicles lined by simple cubical epithelium and filled with watery colloid. The epithelium rests on a poorly developed basement membrane, outside which is an immense capillary network. The colloid is of homogeneous appearance.

Cells of two types are found lining the vesicles, chief cells and parafollicular (or 'C' or light) cells. The majority are chief cells which have a basophilic cytoplasm and produce the colloid, which contains the hormones thyroxin and tri-iodothyronine. These are transferred to the blood stream by pinocytosis on the part of the chief cells. The parafollicular cells are larger and paler than the chief cells and lie singly or in pairs amongst the chief cells. They produce the hormone thyrocalcitonin.

The parathyroid glands
These glands, usually four in number, lie embedded in the back of the thyroid gland. The glands are composed of densely packed epithelial cells with a rich network of capillaries between. The epithelial cells are of two types in man, principal and oxyphil cells. The principal cells are the majority type, and are of small size with a basophilic cytoplasm. They produce the parathyroid hormone. The oxyphil cells are larger than the principal cells and have a pale eosinophilic cytoplasm. They lie in clumps. Their function is unknown.

THE ADRENAL GLANDS

These paired glands lie in the abdominal cavity, one at the upper pole of each kidney. They consist of an outer cortex and an inner medulla of widely divergent origin and function.

The adrenal cortex is composed of epithelial cells arranged in three zones: an outer zona glomerulosa, a middle zona fasciculata and an inner zona reticularis. The boundaries between adjacent zones are not clear cut. The zona glomerulosa consists of elongated basophilic cells arranged in a series of arches not unlike a Roman aqueduct. Capillaries lie between the cells, which are the source of the mineralocorticoids (aldosterone and deoxycorticosterone). The zona fasciculata forms the bulk of the cortex. It is composed of polyhedral cells arranged in long columns with elongated capillaries between. The cells are rich in lipid droplets and in the usual histological section the cells look foamy due to dissolution of the lipid. The cells of this and the next zone produce the glucocorticoids (cortisone and cortisol). The zona reticularis is composed of polyhedral cells arrayed in anastomosing columns. The cells contain some lipid but considerably less than the cells of the zona fasciculata. The innermost part of the zona reticularis contains many degenerative cells, with pycnotic nuclei.

The adrenal medulla consists of clusters of polyhedral cells which produce both adrenaline and nor-adrenaline, surrounded by blood capillaries. The cells are of two types, those which store adrenaline and those which store nor-adrenaline. They are present in numbers that are approximately one nor-adrenaline-storing cell to every four adrenaline-storing cells. Both types, after fixation in potassium bichromate, have fine dark brown cytoplasmic granules and are then said to exhibit the chromaffin reaction. Sympathetic ganglion cells occur singly or in small groups amongst the chromaffin cells.

THE PITUITARY GLAND

The pituitary gland, or hypophysis cerebri is composed partly of epithelial tissue (the adenohypophysis) and partly of nervous tissue (the neurohypophysis). The gland is suspended by a stalk from the floor of the third ventricle.

The adenohypophysis
The adenohypophysis is derived from Rathke's pouch, an upgrowth of stomatodaeal ectoderm. It is composed of the pars anterior, pars intermedia and pars tuberalis.

The pars anterior This is the largest part of the gland. It consists of epithelial cells clustered around capillaries. The epithelial cells are of three types. The acidophils or α-chromophils have eosinophilic cytoplasmic granules. They secrete growth hormone and lactogenic hormone. The second type is the basophil or ß-chromophil. These cells have basophilic cytoplasmic granules and can be divided into two subclasses: the beta basophil is aldehyde fuchsin-positive and produces thyrotropic hormone. The delta basophil is aldehyde fuchsin-negative and elaborates the gonadotrophins, F.S.H and L.H. The third cell type in the pars anterior is the chromophobe, which is agranular. It may be a degranulated chromophil, or a stem cell capable of differentiating into a chromophil, or both.

The pars intermedia The epithelial cells of the pars intermedia are polygonal in outline and have basophil granules in their cytoplasm. They are often arranged around colloid-filled vesicles in a manner highly reminiscent of the thyroid gland. The pars intermedia blends off into the pars anterior round the sides of the stalk: it constitutes only a small portion of the pituitary. Melanocyte-stimulating hormone is produced in the pars intermedia.

The pars tuberalis This is also but a small part of the pituitary. It consists of a collar of epithelial cells surrounding the stalk of the pituitary. The cells are arranged in long columns with elongated capillaries between. The pars tuberalis is the most vascular portion of the pituitary. Its constituent cells are cuboidal, agranular or finely granular. They are arranged often around vesicles filled with a colloid-like material. The function of the pars tuberalis is unknown.

The neurohypophysis
This is composed of the eminentia medialis of the tuber cinereum, the infundibular stalk and the infundibular process (or pars nervosa). It arises as a downgrowth from the diencephalic portion of the prosencephalic vesicle. It is composed of large numbers of non-myelinated nerve fibres and some neuroglial cells known as pituicytes, i.e. it is composed of white matter. The nerve fibres are derived in large measure from the cells of the supra-optic and paraventricular nuclei in the hypothalamus, and the nerve terminals end in close apposition to the capillaries of the pars nervosa. The hormones of the pars nervosa, oxytocin and vasopressin are not produced, but merely stored and then liberated into the

continued

180 *Thyroid gland (H & E)* The parenchyma of the gland is arranged as a cubical epithelium enclosing vesicles filled with homogeneous colloid.

181 *Thyroid gland (H & E)* High power of **180**. Many capillaries (A) lined by endothelium (B) lie in the immediate vicinity of the vesicles.

182 *Thyroid gland (H & E)* Groups of parafollicular or clear cells (*arrowed*) lie in the wall of this follicle. They are larger than, and stain less intensely than, the chief cells.

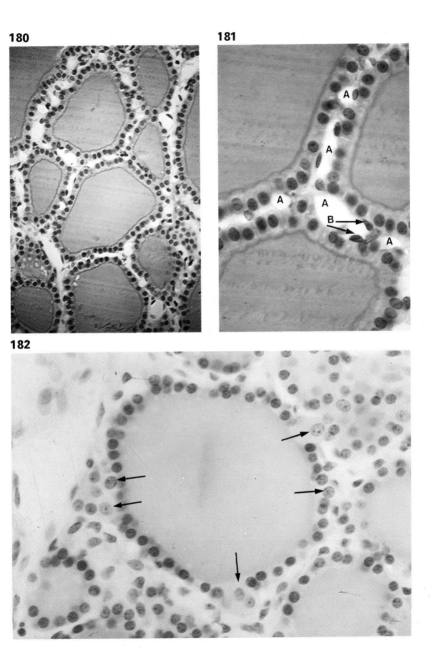

blood stream there. They are elaborated in the cell bodies of the hypothalamic nuclei and track down the axons in the form of membrane-bound granules, as seen with the electron microscope. Localised accumulations of these in grossly expanded regions of the axons would appear without doubt to correspond with the Herring bodies, chrome-alum-positive spherical masses seen with the light microscope. The neuroglial cells or pituicytes of the pars nervosa provide an investment for the axons in the form of slender cytoplasmic processes pervading their midst: the pituicytes may also subserve other functions in connection with the secretory process.

183 *Parathyroid gland (H & E)* The epithelial cells of the gland are mostly chief cells, but an island of oxyphil cells can be seen (*arrows*).

184 *Parathyroid gland (H & E)* High power of **183** to show chief cells (A) and oxyphil cells (B). The oxyphil cells are larger and paler than the chief cells.

185 *Parathyroid gland (Azan)* The island of oxyphil cells (*arrows*) stands out even more prominently with this stain.

186 *Parathyroid gland (Azan)* High power of **185**. The chief cells (A) and oxyphil cells (B) are clearly distinguishable.

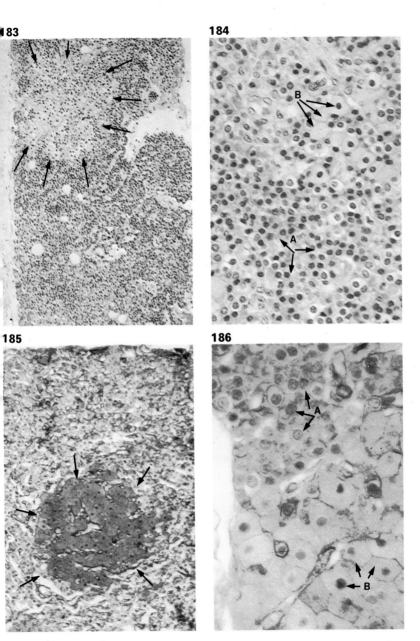

187 *Adrenal gland (Azan)* The collagenous capsule is seen at A. The adrenal cortex is divisible into an outer zona glomerulosa (B), a middle and extensive zona fasciculata (C), and an inner zona reticularis (D). The adrenal medulla lies at E.

188 *Adrenal cortex (H & E)* The zona glomerulosa occupies the upper half of the field. It is composed of cells arranged in arches. The lower half of the picture shows the pale vacuolated cells of the outer fasciculata to be arranged in long columns separated by capillaries.

189 *Adrenal cortex (H & E)* The inner part of the zona fasciculata is here shown. The cells stain darkly but are arranged in long columns with capillaries between.

190 *Adrenal cortex (H & E)* The zona reticularis is shown and is composed of anastomosing columns of epithelial cells, with a rich network of capillary spaces between.

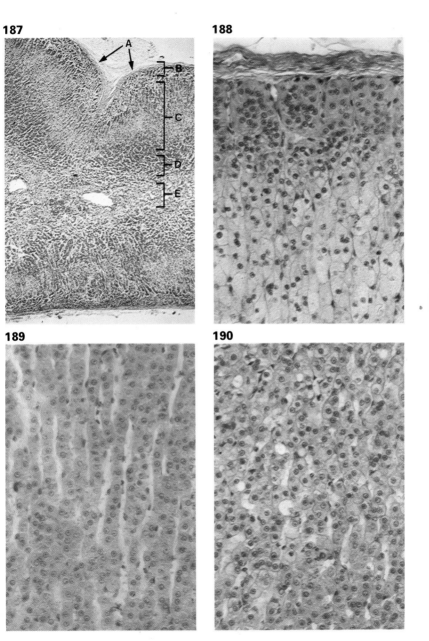

113

191 *Adrenal medulla (H & E)* The medulla of the adrenal gland is composed of clusters of epithelial cells separated by capillaries. The adrenaline and nor-adrenaline storing cells are not differentiated by this stain.

192 *Adrenal medulla (Haematoxylin)* The adrenaline storing cells (A) can be distinguished from the nor-adrenaline storing cells (B) after fixation in glutaraldehyde and dichromate.

193 *The pituitary gland (H & E)* This low power view of a monkey pituitary shows the several parts of the gland. The pars anterior (A) is the largest part of the gland. The lumen of Rathke's pouch is seen at B. The pars intermedia (C) and pars tuberalis (D) are the other portions of the adenohypophysis. The pars nervosa (E) is part of the neurohypophysis. The infundibulum and the third ventricle lie at F and G.

194 *Pituitary gland, pars tuberalis (H & E)* High power view of the pars tuberalis from **193**. This part of the adenohypophysis is composed of small basophil epithelial cells often surrounding colloid-filled vesicles.

195 *Pituitary gland, pars tuberalis (H & E)* High power of **194** to show several vesicles with colloid in the lumen (*arrows*).

191

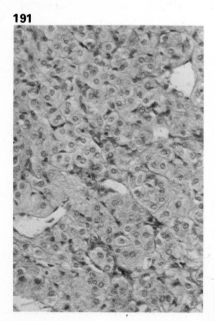

192

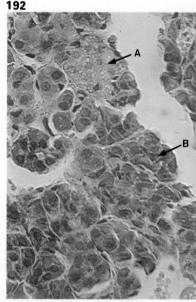

193

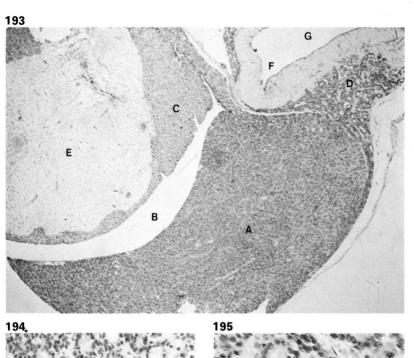

194   **195**

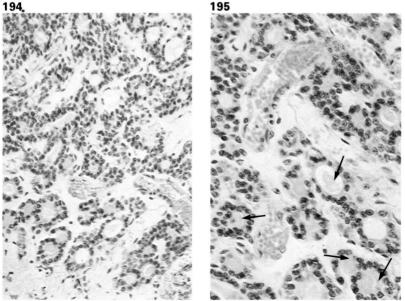

196 *Pituitary gland, pars intermedia (H & E)* High power of a field from **193** to show the small basophil cells of the pars intermedia. Some colloid-filled vesicles are also present (*arrows*).

197 *Pituitary gland, pars intermedia (Gomori)* This human preparation shows that some acidophilic cells (*arrowed*) lie amongst the basophilic cells. A large colloid-filled vesicle occupies the bottom of the field.

198 *Pituitary gland, pars nervosa (H & E)* High power field from **193**. The pars nervosa is composed of white matter—i.e. nerve fibres and neuroglial cells (pituicytes).

199 *Pituitary gland, pars nervosa* In this preparation red blood cells are bright red and neurosecretory material is bright blue. The latter is seen to be para-capillary in distribution.

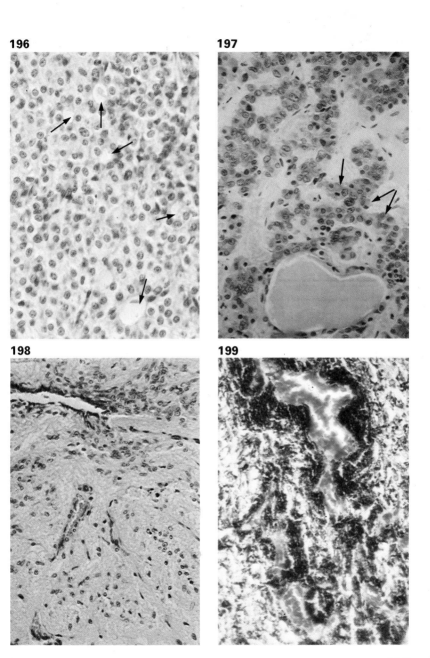

200 *Pituitary gland, pars anterior (H & E)* High power of a field from **193**. Cells with acidophilic cytoplasm (A) and cells with basophilic cytoplasm (B) are in clumps separated by capillaries (C).

201 *Pituitary gland, pars anterior (H & E)* This human preparation shows the same arrangement as in the monkey (**200**).

202 *Pituitary gland, pars anterior (Gomori)* Human pituitary to show acidophils (A) stained red, basophils (B) stained blue and colourless chromophobes (C).

203 *Pituitary gland, pars anterior (Azan)* Human pituitary showing acidophils (A) stained brown, basophils (B) stained blue and near colourless chromophobes (C).

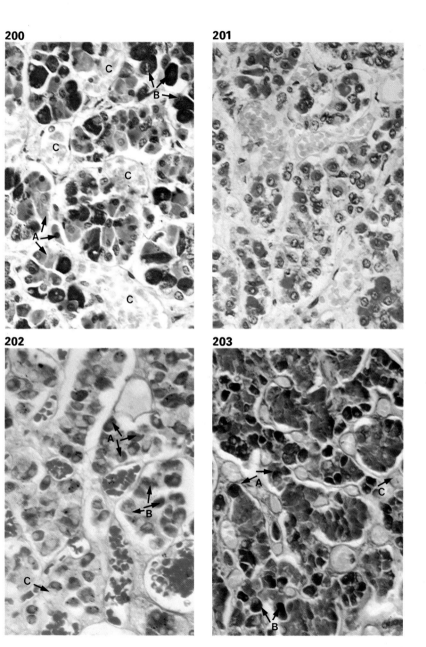

119

The Integument

THE EPIDERMIS AND DERMIS

The skin is composed of an outer epithelial component, the epidermis, and an inner connective tissue component, the dermis or corium. The dermo-epidermal junction is scalloped like an egg-box. Below the dermis is the subcutis, a layer of loose connective tissue connecting the skin with the superficial fascia.

The epidermis
The epidermis consists of stratified squamous epithelium of the keratinising variety. The strata of, and successive changes undergone by the keratinising cells have been described in the chapter on epithelium. Scattered near the basement membrane of the epidermis are to be found the clear cells, so-called because they lack the basophilia and tonofibril complement characteristic of the adjacent cells of the stratum germinitivum, and which therefore stand out in H & E preparations because of their lack of staining. They are of stellate outline and of two types:

Pigment-producing cells or melanoblasts. These produce the pigment melanin which has a protective function. The melanin they produce is liberated and ingested by the cells in the stratum germinitivum and by the deepest cells in the stratum spinosum.

Cells of Langerhans. These are also dendritic and can be demonstrated by impregnation with gold salts. They possess ultrastructural characteristics (deeply indented nuclei and unique cytoplasmic granules) which allow a distinction to be drawn between them and melanoblasts. Their function is unknown.

The dermis
This is composed of connective tissue with nervous and vascular elements, and the glands and hairs of the skin lie embedded in its substance. It can be subdivided into an outer half, the papillary layer and an inner half, the reticular layer. The papillary layer of the dermis is composed of a loose connective tissue containing some reticular fibres. The reticular layer of the dermis is composed of dense irregular connective tissue. Where epithelial structures such as sweat glands and hair follicles extend down into the reticular layer they carry over an investment of loose connective tissue from the superficial zone of the dermis. Smooth muscle is present in the dermis of the penis and scrotum and the areola of the nipple. Skeletal muscle (of facial expression) is found in the dermis of the face and scalp.

The blood vessels of the skin
The epidermis is avascular. There is a network (rete cutaneum) of large arteries and veins at the boundary between dermis and subcutis. From this plexus vessels pass into the dermis, pursuing a curved course. A second plexus, the rete subpapillare is to be found in the superficial reach of the reticular layer. A third

plexus lies at the junction of the reticular and papillary layers: capillary loops pass from this plexus into the dermal papillae. The dermis also contains a rich lymphatic plexus which begins in the dermal papillae as blind capillaries and ends in large valved subdermal lymph vessels.

The nerves of the skin

Naked nerve terminals ramify amongst the epithelial cells of the epidermis. Naked nerve terminals occur in the dermis also, especially around the glands and hair follicles. A rich plexus of nerves occurs throughout the dermis. The fibres are myelinated except in the region immediately deep to the epidermis where they are non-myelinated. Encapsulated nerve endings of two types also occur: the corpuscles of Meissner and the Pacinian corpuscles.

Corpuscles of Meissner These touch receptors lie in the dermal papillae. They are ovoids of some $40 \times 100\mu$ with their long axis at right angles to the surface. They have a thin connective tissue capsule which passes into the interior of the corpuscle dividing it into lobules within which are modified connective tissue cells of conical shape whose base rests on the side wall of, and whose apices project into the interior of the corpuscle. A myelinated nerve fibre enters the corpuscle on its deep aspect and zig-zags its way between the connective tissue cells towards the surface, branching as it does so. With the electron microscope the nerve terminal is seen to make synaptic connections with the connective tissue cells of the corpuscle.

The Pacinian corpuscles These macroscopic entities are several millimetres across and lie in the subcutis. They act as pressure receptors. The corpuscle is spherical or ovoid and on section is not unlike a divided onion in appearance, being composed of an outer bulb of some 30 concentrically-arranged and highly attenuated connective tissue cells with fluid-filled spaces between. The core or inner bulb of the corpuscle is granular when viewed with the light microscope but under the electron microscope is seen to be composed also of concentric connective tissue cells. A medullated nerve fibre enters the corpuscle on its deep aspect and penetrates the successive lamellae to reach the inner bulb where it terminates. The nerve fibre loses its myelin sheath and its Schwann cell sheath as it penetrates the circumferential lamellae. The nerve terminal in the inner bulb is seen with the electron microscope to have a remarkable palisade of radially-arranged mitochondria at its circumference.

THE GLANDS OF THE SKIN

Exocrine glands of three types occur in the skin: sweat glands, 'apocrine' glands and sebaceous glands.

Sweat glands

These are simple coiled tubular glands. The secretory part of the gland is coiled and lies either in the subcutis or in the reticular layer of the dermis. The duct portion of the gland is straight in its course through the dermis but corkscrews its way through the epidermis.

The secretory portion of the sweat gland is lined by pseudo-stratified columnar epithelium. Myo-epithelial cells are present. The secretory cells are of two types named according to their E.M. appearance and are present in numbers that are approximately equal. The 'dark' cells present a broad surface towards the lumen and are narrow basally. They have prominent periodic acid-Schiff positive apical granules and produce the mucin component of sweat. The 'clear' cells produce the watery component of sweat, and lie towards the periphery of the tubule. They have narrow apices and broad bases. Intercellular canaliculi lined by microvilli are seen between them in electron micrographs.

The intra-dermal portion of the duct of the gland is lined by stratified cubical epithelium. There is evidence from E.M. studies that the lining cells of the duct modify the secretion as it passes to the surface. The coiled intra-epidermal portion of the duct is lined by the cells of the successive strata of the epidermis.

The 'apocrine' glands

These occur in the axilla, groin, and external genital region. They differ from conventional sweat glands in that they are much larger, and become fully differentiated only after puberty. They are similar in that they are simple coiled tubuloalveolar glands subdivisible into a secretory and a duct portion, and possess myoepithelial cells in the former.

The secretory segment is lined by a simple epithelium which ranges from squamous to columnar in type. Only one cell type is present. It possesses prominent periodic acid Schiff-positive granules in its apical cytoplasm. With the electron microscope these are seen to be modified mitochondria. Prominent apical cytoplasmic pseudopodia are often seen in the cells and the older histologists assumed that these became pinched-off to form the secretion of the gland, hence the 'apocrine' tag.

The duct of the gland is lined by stratified cubical epithelium. The ceruminous glands of the external auditory meatus and the glands of Moll of the eyelid have a morphology similar to that of the apocrine glands.

The sebaceous glands

These glands lie in the papillary layer of the dermis and are simple or, rarely, branched alveolar glands. They open invariably into the lumen of a hair follicle except at the margins of the lips, the areola and the labia minora where they open directly onto the skin surface. They may attain a size of some 2mm in diameter.

The sebaceous gland is no more than a bag of cells and the secretion (sebum) of the gland is composed of degenerate cells desquamated from the lining of the bag—i.e. the gland secretes by the holocrine method. The wall of the gland is composed of cells continuous with the cells of the stratum germinitivum of the outer epithelial root sheath of the associated hair follicle. The cellular contents of the bag show progressive changes indicative of degeneration the further they are found from the wall of the alveolus. These changes are:

Decrease in cytoplasmic basophilia.　　　　*Increase in nuclear pycnosis.*

Increase in cell size.　　　　*Increase in content of cytoplasmic lipid.*

THE HAIRS

Hairs are epithelial derivatives composed of a shaft, which is the part above the skin surface and a root which is embedded in the skin. The lower end of the root is expanded to form the hair bulb, the deep extremity of which is indented by a goblet-shaped mass of connective tissue known as the hair papilla. The epithelial investment of the root of the hair is known as the hair follicle.

The hair proper is formed of cornified horny epithelial cells. It is composed from within outwards of medulla, cortex, and cuticle. The medulla comprises two or three rows of epithelial cells which in the hair root are polyhedral in outline. The medullary cells of the hair show evidence of progressive degeneration as they move up the shaft and the medulla eventually peters out. Pigment is found in the medullary cells, the amount decreasing with age. The cortex forms the main bulk of the hair: the epithelial cells of the cortex are cubical in the hair root but scale-like in the shaft. As the cells ascend they acquire increasing numbers of birefringent fibrils in their cytoplasm. The cuticle of the cortex is composed of a series of horny plates arranged like slates on a roof and interdigitating with the scales of the inner epithelial root sheath of the follicle, which are arranged in similar fashion. By this means the hair is anchored in the follicle.

The hair follicle is composed of an inner epithelial root sheath and an outer epithelial root sheath. A connective tissue root sheath lies outside this.

The inner epithelial root sheath is composed of three rows of epithelial cells, named from within outwards the cuticle of the inner root sheath, the layer of Huxley, and the layer of Henlé. Like the hair, this root sheath grows by replacement from the dividing cells in the bulb below and the inner epithelial root sheath is present only as far as the opening into the follicle of the sebaceous gland: here the now degenerate epithelial cells of the sheath are desquamated into the lumen of the follicle.

The outer epithelial root sheath is composed of the stratum germinitivum and stratum spinosum of the epidermis which dips into the follicle. It is well developed superficially but in the depths of the follicle becomes progressively less well defined and finally peters out on the surface of the hair bulb. The connective tissue root sheath is composed of both circular and longitudinal collagen fibres from the dermis: it is separated from the outer epithelial root sheath by the basement membrane of the epithelium.

THE NAILS

These protective devices are epithelial derivatives composed of a superficial hard portion, the nail body, and a deep soft part, the nail bed. The proximal part of the nail is buried in the dermis and is known as the nail root. Growth of the nail results from mitotic activity of the cells in the root. Newly-formed nail is opaque and this accounts for the lunula or half-moon of the nail.

The body of the nail is analagous with the stratum corneum of unmodified epidermis and is composed of nucleated horny plates. The nail bed consists of the stratum spinosum and stratum germinitivum of the epidermis. The stratum granulosum is not represented in the nail and ends abruptly at the nail margin.

The stratum corneum of the epidermis adjacent to the nail is thickened to form the eponychium (round the nail margins) and the hyponychium (below the free margin of the nail). The dermo-epidermo junction in the nail takes the form of longitudinal ridges running proximo-distally.

---

204 *Thick, hairless skin (H & E)* The skin is composed of a superficial epithelial component, the epidermis (A), and a deeper connective tissue component, the dermis, which is subdivisible in turn into a superficial papillary layer (B) and a deep reticular layer (C). Sweat glands (D) lie in the last layer.

205 *Epidermis of thick skin (H & E)* High power of a field from **204** to show the epidermis. For explanation see **12**.

206 *Epidermis of skin (H & E)* In this field several clear cells (*arrows*) are to be seen in the deeper reaches of the epidermis.

207 *Epidermis of skin (H & E)* This preparation is taken from an individual of heavy pigmentation. The pigment (melanin) lies in the cells of the stratum germinitivum and in the deeper cells of the stratum spinosum.

204

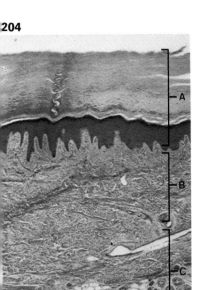

205

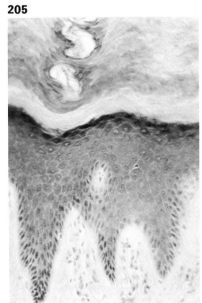

206

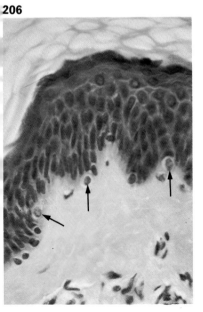

207

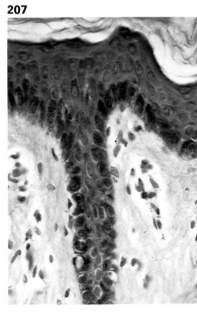

208 *Dermis of skin (H & E)* High power of a field from **204**. The papillary layer is shown and is seen to be composed of loose connective tissue investing a network of blood vessels and nerves (A). An epidermal papilla is seen at B.

209 *Blood vessels of skin, injected preparation* The rete cutaneum (A) lies at the junction of dermis and subcutis. The rete subpapillare (B) lies in the reticular layer of the dermis. A smaller plexus (C) is found in the papillary layer of the dermis.

210 *Palmar skin (H & E)* The sweat glands (A) lie in the dermis (B) and in the subcutis (C). The Pacinian corpuscles (D) lie in the subcutis, which is composed mainly of adipose tissue.

208

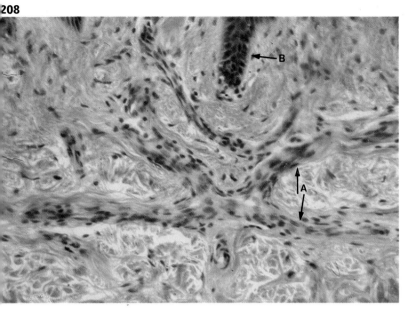

209

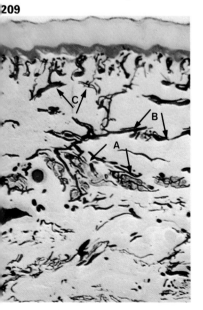

210

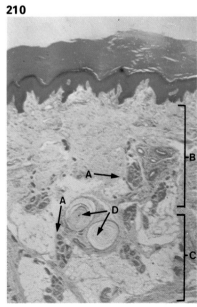

211 *Skin, corpuscles of Meissner (H & E)* Two corpuscles lie in this field (*arrows*). They are strongly eosinophilic ovoids composed of connective tissue cells investing a nerve terminal: the latter is not seen with this stain.

212 *Skin, corpuscle of Meissner (Silver)* The nerve fibre is seen zig-zagging its way through the interior of the corpuscle after silver staining.

213 *Skin, Pacinian corpuscle (H & E)* The corpuscle is composed of an outer bulb (A) and an inner bulb (B) of attenuated connective tissue cells. The encapsulated nerve terminal is not seen with this stain.

214 *Sweat glands of skin (H & E)* High power of a field from **204** to show the coiled portion of a sweat gland.

215 *Sweat glands of skin (H & E)* The secretory segment (A) is lined by pseudo-stratified columnar epithelium. The dark and clear cells are not differentiated by this stain. The duct segment (B) is lined by stratified cubical epithelium. Myoepithelial cell nuclei (C) are seen in the secretory segment.

211

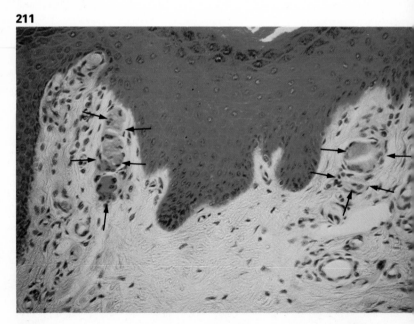

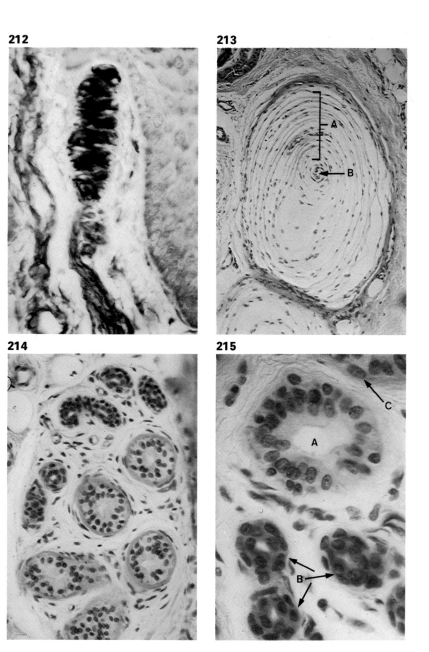

212

213

A

B

214

215

A

C

B

129

216 *Sweat gland of skin (H & E)* The junction between secretory segment (A) and duct segment (B) is abrupt (*arrows*).

217 *Duct of sweat gland (H & E)* The intra-epidermal portion of the duct is lined by the cells of the successive strata of the epidermis, through which it corkscrews its way to the surface.

218 *'Apocrine' glands of skin (H & E)* Skin from mons veneris of a female showing modified sweat glands. From left to right are squamous secretory segment, cubical secretory segment, ducts and columnar secretory segment.

219 *'Apocrine' glands of skin (H & E)* High power view of columnar secretory segment in transverse section. The lining is simple columnar and the cells possess apical pseudopodia.

220 *'Apocrine' glands of skin (H & E)* High power view of columnar-epithelial lined secretory segment in longitudinal section. The apical pseudo-podia are again conspicuous and led the older histologists to conclude that the cells secreted by the 'apocrine' method.

216

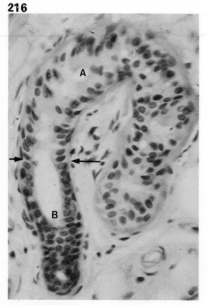

217

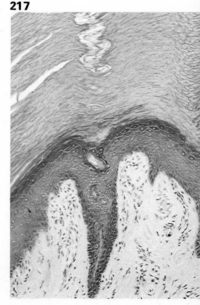

218

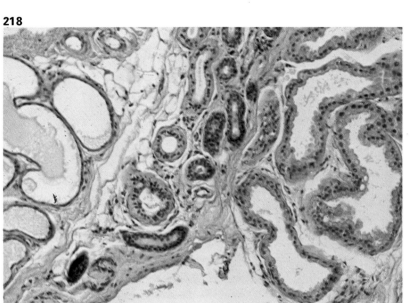

219

220

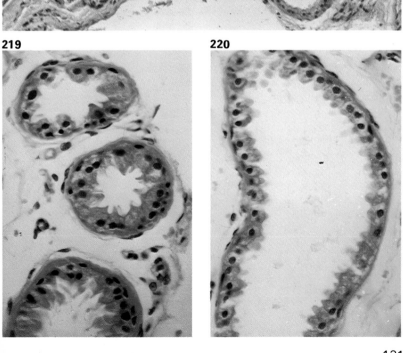

221 *Sebaceous glands of skin (H & E)* The sebaceous glands (A) are almost universally associated with hair follicles (B). Arrectores pilorum muscles are present (C).

222 *Sebaceous glands of skin (H & E)* A single hair follicle (A) and its group of associated sebaceous glands (B) are seen.

223 *Sebaceous glands of skin (H & E)* The cells within the lumen of the gland show evidence of progressive degenerative change and increase in size as they move towards the surface (*top*).

224 *Sebaceous glands of skin (H & E)* The intimate relationship between an arrector pili muscle (A) and the sebaceous gland (B) is here illustrated.

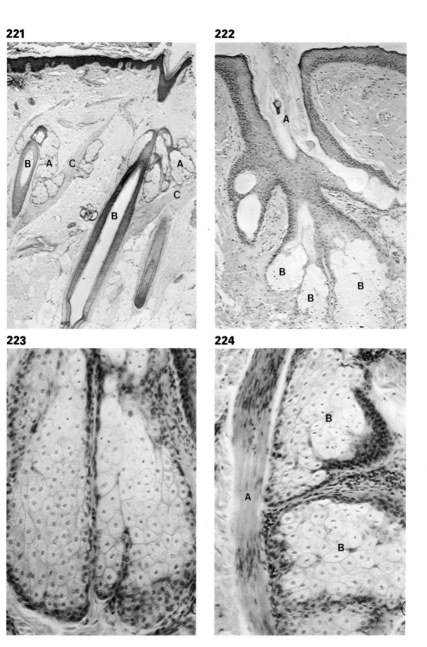

221

222

223

224

133

225 *LS hair follicle (H & E)* The epidermis is seen at A. The hair follicle (B) is cut longitudinally. The hair bulb lies at C. A sebaceous gland (D) opens into the superficial part of the follicle.

226 *LS hair follicle (H & E)* High power of the hair bulb in **225**. The undifferentiated cells of the bulb lie at A. The commencement of the root of the hair is at B. The inner epithelial (C) and outer epithelial (D) root sheaths are well shown. The connective tissue root sheath lies at E.

227 *LS hair follicle (H & E)* High power of the middle third of the hair follicle in **225**. The hair root (A) is invested by the inner epithelial root sheath (B), the outer epithelial root sheath (C) and the connective tissue root sheath (D).

228 *LS hair follicle (H & E)* High power view of the superficial one-third of the hair follicle in **225**. The hair root (A) is now invested by an attenuated inner epithelial root sheath (B) and an expanding outer epithelial root sheath (C). The connective tissue root sheath is seen at D.

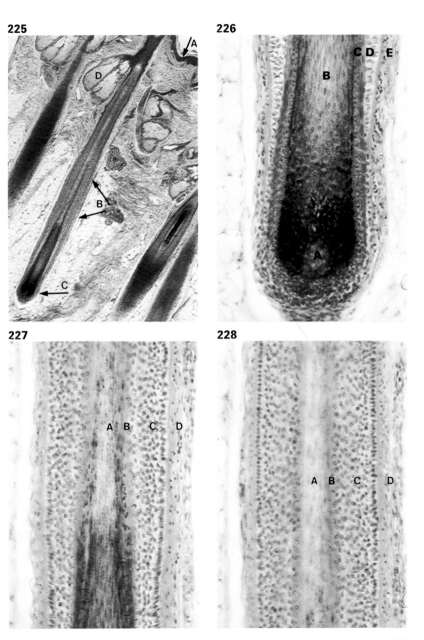

135

229 *TS hair follicle (H & OGE)* The hair root (A) is sectioned at a deep level since the inner epithelial root sheath (B) is well developed. The outer epithelial root sheath is at C and the connective tissue root sheath at D.

230 *TS hair follicle (H & E)* The hair root (A) is sectioned at an intermediate level since the inner epithelial root sheath (B) is now less well defined whilst the outer epithelial root sheath (C) is well developed. The connective tissue root sheath is again at D.

231 *TS hair follicle (H & E)* The follicle (A) is sectioned at the level of the opening of the sebaceous gland (B).

232 *TS hair follicle (H & E)* The most superficial part of the follicle (A) is lined by the cornified epidermis (B) which here forms the outer epithelial root sheath.

233 *Hair follicle, attachment of arrector pili (H & OGE)* The smooth muscle bundle of the arrector pili (A) is attached to the connective tissue root sheath (B) of the hair follicle. The outer epithelial root sheath (C) is invariably swollen at the point of attachment.

229

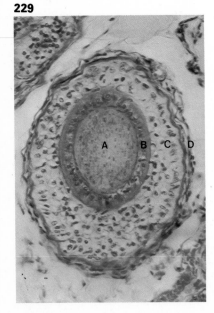

230

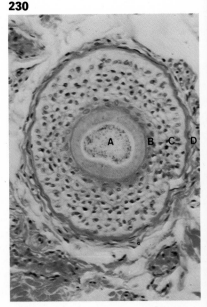

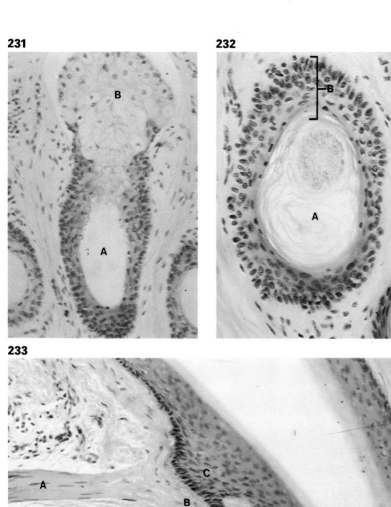

231

232

233

137

234 *TS nail (H & OGE)* The terminal phalanx of the finger is at A. The nail (B) is flanked by eponychium (C).

235 *TS nail (H & OGE)* High power view of **234**. The nail body (A) is composed of nucleated horny plates. The nail bed (B) is composed of stratum spinosum and stratum germinitivum. The proximo-distally disposed dermal ridges lie at C.

236 *TS nail (H & OGE)* High power of **234** to show the nail margin and the eponychium. The stratum granulosum is not represented in the nail and terminates at A.

237 *LS nail (H & E)* The nail bed lies at A, the eponychium is seen at B and the nail body is at C.

234

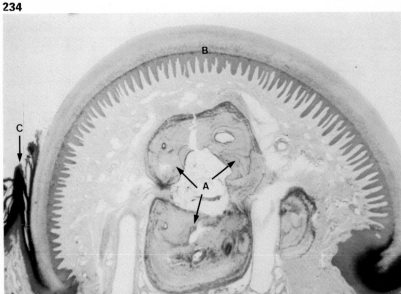

235

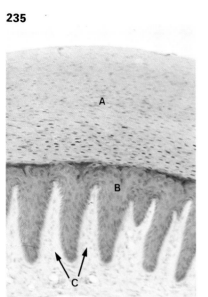

236

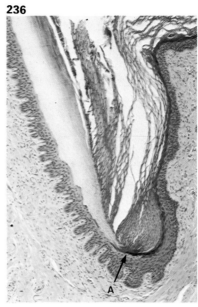

237

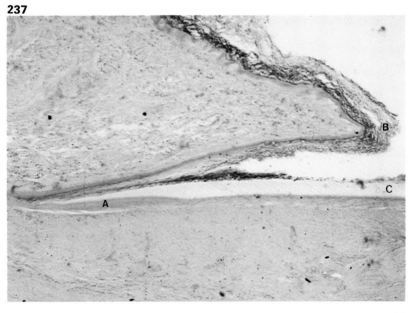

The Alimentary Tract

THE ORAL CAVITY

The oral cavity extends from the muco-cutaneous junction of the lip anteriorly to the oropharyngeal isthmus posteriorly. It is lined by a mucous membrane. The epithelium is stratified squamous, mucous membrane variety, the superficial cells of which desquamate into the saliva in large numbers. The epithelium is non-cornified except on the dorsum of the tongue. Beneath the epithelium is loose connective tissue known as the corium or lamina propria. The boundary between epithelium and corium may be plane or scalloped. The blood vessels are arranged in a manner akin to that of skin—i.e. there is a submucous plexus of large vessels, a plexus of smaller vessels in the deeper part of the corium and capillary loops in the superficial part of the corium. There is also a rich submucous plexus of nerves derived from the trigeminal nerve. This plexus in turn supports a finer subepithelial plexus which sends fibres to the taste buds and naked fibres into the lining epithelium. All the muscle of the oral cavity is of the skeletal variety.

The teeth
These arise in part from epithelium (viz the enamel) and in part from connective tissue (viz the dentine, cementum, pulp cavity and periodontal membrane). A tooth consists of a crown, which projects above gum level, and a root which is embedded below gum level in the alveolar bone of mandible or maxilla. The neck of the tooth lies at the junction of root and crown.

The crown of the tooth is composed of dentine covered on its surface by enamel and enclosing the superficial part of the pulp cavity. The root of the tooth is composed of dentine covered by cementum and enclosing the deep part of the pulp cavity.

The pulp cavity The pulp cavity is composed of vascular loose connective tissue continuous at the apex of the root with the loose connective tissue of the gum; it carries blood vessels and nerves. Around the circumference of the pulp cavity are to be found the odontoblasts which were responsible for the manufacture of the dentine and which send long processes of cytoplasm into its substance.

The enamel As with all other epithelia enamel is avascular. It is composed of hexagonal prisms which represent the modified basal regions of the ameloblast cells which at one time lay on its surface but which become eroded as the tooth erupts. Enamel is the hardest tissue in the body, being 96% inorganic.

Dentine Dentine is also a very hard tissue and its proportions ($\frac{1}{3}$ organic, $\frac{2}{3}$ inorganic) are very akin to those of bone. Dentine is devoid of cell bodies, and is avascular. Dentine is composed of elongated dentinal tubules which branch and anastomose and contain odontoblast cytoplasmic processes bathed in extra-cellular fluid. The hard calcified inorganic dentinal matrix surrounds the tubules. This matrix is laid down in spheres and becomes calcified afterwards. The intervals between the spheres are known as interglobular spaces. These are large in the crown. In the root they are smaller and arranged in a vertical row in the peripheral dentine where they are known as Tomes' granular layer.

The cementum This covers the outer aspect of the dentine of the root of the tooth. It is composed of compact bone but devoid of the Haversian systems normally present in such bone. It may be cellular or acellular. In the former, the osteocytes lie in lacunae surrounded by canaliculi into the proximal ends of which they send cytoplasmic projections.

The periodontal membrane The periodontal membrane is composed of collagen bundles embedded at one extremity in the cementum and at the other end in the alveolar bone. It holds the tooth anchored in its socket.

THE SALIVARY GLANDS

These occur in the oral cavity in two forms: as widespread yet localised collections in the corium or submucosa of all parts of the mouth, and as three larger circumscribed paired masses lying some distance from the buccal cavity and opening into it by elongated ducts. These are the parotid, submandibular (or submaxillary) and sublingual salivary glands.

Acini
All salivary glands are of the compound tubulo-acinar form. The acini are of three types: mucous, serous and mixed.

Mucous acini These are spherical or ovoid tubules lined by truncated pyramidal cells. The nucleus is usually flattened against the base of the cells. The supranuclear cytoplasm is pale due to its complement of many large mucin droplets. Myoepithelial cells are present.

Serous acini These are rather smaller spherical tubules lined by truncated pyramidal cells. The nucleus is spherical and located near the middle of the cell. The apical cytoplasm contains eosinophilic zymogen granules which are the forerunners of the enzyme ptyalase. Myoepithelial cells are also present.

Mixed acini These are terminal secretory segments composed of a mucous acinus with a serous demilune or crescent on its distal aspect. The secretion of the serous cells reaches the lumen by passing through intercellular canaliculi between the mucous cells.

Ducts

The major salivary glands may exhibit ducts of three types:

Intercalated ducts These have a cross-sectional diameter which is less than that of an acinus. They are, when present, the earliest and smallest portion of the duct system and are lined by a simple cubical epithelium. They are abundant only in glands of the pure serous type—i.e. in the parotid (and pancreas and lacrimal glands, as will be seen later). The intercalated ducts open into the striated intralobular ducts.

Striated intralobular ducts These have a cross-sectional diameter equivalent to or marginally greater than that of an acinus. They are abundant in all three oral salivary glands, are easily recognisable within the substance of the lobule and are lined by a simple low columnar epithelium. The basal region of the cells exhibits many infoldings of the plasma membrane with elongated mitochondria between. A basal striation is by this means imparted to the cell. These lead to the interlobular ducts.

Interlobular ducts These lie in the connective tissue septa between the lobules of the gland and join up to form the main secretory duct or ducts of the gland and which open into the buccal cavity. They are lined by pseudostratified columnar epithelium, and goblet cells may be present.

The parotid gland is composed exclusively of serous acini and possesses intercalated, intralobular and interlobular ducts. The sublingual gland is composed of serous acini, mucous acini and mixed acini. Intercalated ducts are uncommon in the gland since they will be found only in the pure mucous and serous segments. The mixed acini of the gland open into intralobular ducts directly. Interlobular ducts are present. The submandibular gland is pre-dominantly serous although some of the acini are mixed. Intercalated ducts are found in the pure serous segments. Intralobular and interlobular ducts are found.

The salivary glands of the other parts of the buccal cavity are as follows:

Labial   Mucous acini

Buccal—i.e. cheek   Mucous and serous acini

Anterior tongue   Mucous with serous crescents

Posterior tongue   1) Associated with circumvallate papil-
                                   lae are serous acini
                                   2) At the root of the tongue are mucous
                                   acini

Palatine glands   Mucous acini

THE TONGUE

This organ is composed of skeletal muscle covered by a mucous membrane. The epithelium of the mucosa is stratified squamous epithelium of the mucous membrane type, and is non-keratinised except on the anterior part of the dorsum. The corium has papillary projections into the epithelium and is firmly adherent to the underlying muscle so that the mucosa of the tongue is immoveable.

The tongue is subdivisible anatomically, embryologically and histologically into an anterior two-thirds and a posterior one-third. The demarcating line is seen as a groove, the sulcus limitans, on the dorsum of the tongue. The groove is V-shaped with the apex posteriorly. Anterior to the sulcus the dorsum of the tongue is rough, but behind it is smooth and shiny as are the sides and underside of the tongue. The roughness is due to the presence of the lingual papillae which are of three types: filiform, fungiform and circumvallate.

Filiform papillae

These are the smallest and most numerous of the papillae, and are arranged in rows which, near the sulcus are parallel to the sulcus but which near the front of the tongue run transversely. They are of conical shape with a covering of scaly keratinised epithelial cells; the cells have progressed to cornification without passing through the intermediary of a stratum granulosum however. These papillae appear to subserve a purely mechanical function.

The fungiform papillae

These are of pin-head size, of red colour and mushroom shape. They are scattered at random over the dorsum of the tongue. The covering epithelium is thin and non-keratinised. Some taste buds are present on the side walls. The papillae have a core of connective tissue.

The circumvallate papillae

These number some 12–20 and lie just in front of the sulcus limitans. Each is about the size of the head of a match and is surrounded by a trench, outside which is a circular ridge. Many taste buds lie in the side wall of both papilla and trench. The covering epithelium is non-keratinised. The connective tissue core is extensive. Deep to the trench are found serous glands (of von Ebner).

Taste buds

These are large barrel-shaped structures embedded in the epithelium. They extend from the basement membrane to the surface and open to the surface at a

143

minute taste pore. They are composed of banana-shaped cells of two types:
Gustatory cells. These have oval darkly-staining nuclei and end superficially in tiny hairs which project from the taste pore.
Sustentacular cells. These have pale, round nuclei.

The mucosa of the posterior third of the tongue is raised into many rounded elevations by masses of lymphoid tissue (lingual tonsil), in the corium. The mucosa is smooth and shiny. A ring of lymphoid tissue surrounds the oro-pharyngeal isthmus in the shape of the lingual tonsil, palatine tonsils and the nasopharyngeal tonsils (or adenoids).

THE LIPS

The lips are covered externally by skin and internally by the mucous membrane of the mouth. At the muco-cutaneous junction (i.e. at the margin of the red part of the lip) there is an abrupt increase in the height of the epithelium. The papillae in the red part of the lip are very deep and vascular. The bulk of the lip is composed of skeletal muscle (orbicularis oris). Hair follicles and sebaceous and sweat glands are found in the skin of the lip. The labial glands lie on the inside and are mucous in type. Sebaceous glands unassociated with hair follicles are also found in the red part of the lip and in the newborn are important for suckling.

THE PHARYNX

This pathway is shared in common by the respiratory and alimentary tracts. The lining epithelium of the upper pharynx is pseudo-stratified ciliated columnar and in the lower pharynx, stratified squamous epithelium of the mucous membrane variety. In the corium are striped muscle, mucous and serous glands and lymphoid tissue in the form either of collections of lymphocytes or as lymphatic nodules. The outer coat is of dense fibro-elastic tissue.

The soft palate
This is covered on its upper aspect by pseudo-stratified ciliated columnar epithelium and on its inferior surface by stratified squamous epithelium of the mucous membrane variety. It has a core of loose connective tissue containing mucous salivary glands and skeletal muscle. Lymphoid tissue in the form of solitary nodules is frequently found just deep to the epithelium.

The palatine tonsils
These are almond-sized projections into the side wall of the pharynx in the interval between the palato-glossal and palato-pharyngeal folds. They are composed of masses of lymphoid tissue in the corium, and covered by stratified squamous epithelium which dips deeply into the tonsillar substance to form the tonsillar crypts. The lymphoid tissue is mainly in the form of nodules whose peripheral cuff of lymphocytes is asymmetrical, being greater on the juxtapharyngeal than on the other aspects of the nodule because the lymphocytes migrate through the overlying epithelium to reach the saliva. In the process the epithelium frequently becomes so heavily infiltrated with lymphocytes as to be almost unrecognisable—i.e. the epithelium is atypical or reticulated, and its protective power is thereby greatly reduced. Lymphatics are present in the tonsil as anywhere else in the body but no filtering mechanism is present. Mucous salivary glands are also found.

THE TUBULAR PORTIONS OF THE GUT

The tubular portions of the gut follow a common pattern in that their wall is composed of four distinct layers, which from within outwards are the mucous coat or mucosa, the submucosa, the muscularis and the serous coat or serosa.

The mucous coat or mucosa is composed of an inner lining epithelium which is columnar except in the oesophagus and terminal part of the anal canal where it is stratified squamous, a muscularis mucosae of smooth muscle, and a corium of loose reticular connective tissue.

The submucosa consists of dense irregular connective tissue. Mucous glands are found here in the upper and lower oesophagus and the duodenum. An autonomic nerve plexus (of Meissner) is also encountered.

The muscularis is composed of an inner layer of circular and an outer layer of longitudinal muscle. The muscle is smooth except in the upper oesophagus and terminal third of the anal canal where it is skeletal. Between the two coats lies another autonomic nerve plexus (of Auerbach).

The serous coat or serosa is composed of loose connective tissue covered externally by the endothelium of the visceral peritoneum. As is to be expected, the endothelium is not present on the intrathoracic portion of the oesophagus nor in the anal canal.

THE OESOPHAGUS

The oesophagus is lined by stratified squamous epithelium of the mucous membrane variety, and it may be keratinised in places, but a stratum granulosum is never seen. No glands are to be found in the corium. The muscularis mucosae is arranged longitudinally.

The submucosa contains mucous glands at the upper and lower ends and opposite the bifurcation of the trachea. They open to the surface by long ducts lined by cubical epithelium.

The muscularis is skeletal in the upper third, mixed in the middle third and smooth in the lower third.

No serosa is to be found except on the lowest inch of the oesophagus where it lies in the peritoneal cavity.

THE STOMACH

This is lined by simple columnar epithelium which dips in to form the gastric pits. The muscularis mucosae is arranged in an inner circular and outer longitudinal layer. The corium contains glands whose nature varies with the region of the stomach. They open into the pits.

The cardiac glands
The cardiac glands are compound tubulo-alveolar mucus-secreting.

The fundic glands
The fundic glands are simple test tube glands lined by a simple columnar epithelium in which four cell types are encountered:

Mucous neck cells. These lie near the top of the gland and contain prominent supra-nuclear granules which stain with mucous stains such as mucicarmine or the periodic acid-Schiff reaction.

Chief or zymogen cells. These are found throughout the length of the gland but are commoner in the lower than the upper half. The cells are of cubical or low columnar form and have cytoplasmic basophilia. They have large granules of zymogen in their apical cytoplasm. The granules are believed to be the forerunners of the enzyme pepsin. The chief cells probably produce 'intrinsic factor' in addition.

The oxyntic or parietal cells. These are large polyhedral eosinophilic cells which lie at the periphery of the gland near the basement membrane and between the bases of the chief cells. They have massive surface infolds and many mitochondria. They secrete hydrochloric acid. They are commoner in the top than the bottom half of the gland.

The argentaffine cells. These can be shown by silver impregnation and almost certainly exist in two different forms. They occur near the bottom of the gland and lie singly or rarely in pairs between the chief cells. They produce 5-hydroxytryptamine.

The pyloric glands
The pyloric glands are simple coiled tubular glands lined by simple columnar epithelium. Only two cell types are present, mucus-secreting cells and argentaffine cells. The mucous cells are probably identical with the mucous neck cells of the fundic glands and the mucous cells of the submucosal glands (of Brünner) of the duodenum.

The submucosa of the stomach has no features peculiar to it; it is composed of dense irregular connective tissue.

The muscularis is usually in three layers—inner oblique, middle circular and outer longitudinal, all of smooth muscle. The middle circular layer is greatly thickened in the pyloric region where it forms the sphincter.

A serous coat is present except along the greater and lesser curvatures.

THE SMALL INTESTINE

This has a lining of simple columnar epithelium with a striated border. Goblet cells are scattered singly here and there. The goblet cells are pale in H & E preparations, and are flask-shaped with a foamy cytoplasm and the nucleus is compressed against the base of the cell. They contain and secrete mucus which can be stained by mucicarmine or the periodic acid-Schiff reaction. The corium is of reticular connective tissue. A muscularis mucosae is present. The small intestine shows adaptations specific for absorption as follows:

The lining epithelial cells have a prominent brush border of microvilli.

The mucosa sends finger-like projections known as villi into the lumen.

The mucosa and submucosa are thrown into folds known as plicae conniventes.

The lining epithelium dips into the corium between the villi to form simple test-tube glands known as the crypts of Lieberkühn. Goblet cells are less common in the crypts than over the villi. Argentaffine cells are found in the crypts. Here one also encounters the Paneth cells. These are basophilic cells scattered singly or in small groups amongst the lining epithelial cells. They have prominent supranuclear granules which stain with certain dyes such as Orange G. They probably produced lysozyme.

The villi are finger-like projections of the mucous membrane and give it a 'pile', like velvet. They are covered externally by the lining epithelium of the gut and have a core of highly cellular loose connective tissue (corium). Strands of muscularis mucosae extend into the villi. In addition each villus possesses a central lymphatic capillary lined by endothelium. This lymph vessel is usually called the central lacteal because its contained lymph is cloudy due to the fact that it contains particles of fat absorbed from the lumen. The central lacteal drains into larger lymph vessels in the submucosa.

The submucosa of the small gut has the same structure as the submucosa elsewhere.

The muscularis is composed of inner circular and outer longitudinal layers of smooth muscle. A serosa is present.

The duodenum and ileum possess special characteristics known as the glands of Brünner and the Peyer's patches respectively.

The glands of Brünner
These mucus-secreting glands lie in the submucosa of the first three parts of the duodenum, but are usually absent from the fourth part.

Peyer's patches

These are large masses of lymphoid tissue ($1\frac{1}{2}$ inch × $\frac{1}{2}$ inch) found on the antimesenteric border of the ileum. Over the patches the villi are present in reduced numbers so the patches stand out as smooth shiny areas because the mucosa elsewhere has a furry appearance due to the villi. The lymphoid tissue is present in the corium of the mucosa in the form of lymph nodules with germinal centres. The lymphoid tissue usually overflows into the submucosa, however, through gaps in the muscularis mucosae.

THE LARGE INTESTINE

This is lined by simple columnar epithelium with a striated border. Goblet cells are present in greater numbers than in the small intestine. Villi are absent but crypts of Lieberkühn are present, so that the mucous membrane is smooth, with pores. The only other differences between the small and large intestines are that the submucosa of the large gut usually contains fat cells and the outer longitudinal layer of the muscularis is in the form of three disconnected bands or taeniae. The appendix and rectum are the only portions of the large gut with a complete outer longitudinal muscle layer. The appendix has lymphoid tissue in the form of nodules with germinal centres in its corium. The lymphoid tissue is found round the complete circumference of the organ.

The anal canal

This can be divided into three parts on the basis of its lining epithelium. The first part is lined by simple columnar epithelium with goblet cells—i.e. by a continuation of rectal epithelium. The other layers of this part of the anal canal are as for the large gut except that no serosa is found.

The intermediate one-third of the anal canal is lined by stratified squamous epithelium of the mucous membrane variety. The muscularis mucosae is now absent but the other layers of the wall are as for the large gut. The inner circular smooth muscle coat is thickened to form the internal sphincter. Modified sweat glands lie in this part of the canal.

The terminal third of the anal canal is lined by hairy skin, with sebaceous glands. The corium contains also circum-anal or hepatoid glands which look like small isolated masses of liver tissue and which open into the hair follicles by short ducts lined by cubical epithelium. Large amounts of skeletal muscle, the external sphincter, are also found here.

THE LIVER AND BILIARY APPARATUS

The liver is the largest gland in the body and its cells secrete by both the endocrine and exocrine methods. The cells are arranged in elongated lobules around a central vein, a tributary of the hepatic vein. The lobules are not sharply demarcated from one another. They are composed of radially-arranged plates of epithelial cells bathed on both surfaces by sinusoids. The lobules are hexagonal in cross-section and in the angles between the lobules will be found the periportal areas, strands of connective tissue containing a branch of the hepatic artery, of the portal vein and bile ducts and lymphatic vessels. The liver is covered by serosa resting on a connective tissue capsule.

The liver parenchyma
The liver cells are large (20–25μ), hexagonal and sometimes binucleate. The nucleus is central, spherical and conspicuous. The cytoplasm is basophilic since liver cells manufacture protein. The cells contain significant deposits of lipid and glycogen. Liver cells do not appear to vary in appearance from one part of the organ to another and each liver cell seems to be capable of carrying out all the functions of the liver. There is no basement membrane between the liver cells and the hepatic sinusoids.

The liver sinusoids
These start at the periphery of the lobule where they receive blood from the hepatic artery and the portal vein, and terminate in the centre of the lobule by opening into the central vein. They are lined by a discontinuous layer of stellate reticulo-endothelial cells (of von Küpffer) but there are many who believe that the lining consists of endothelial cells and reticulo-endothelial cells in admixture. The sinusoids are surrounded by reticular (argyrophil) fibres and an extravascular space (of Disse) lies between them and the liver cells.

The intrahepatic biliary apparatus
The smallest vessels in this system are the bile canaliculi which are elongated localised expansions of the intercellular space between any two adjacent liver cells. As a result they are angular structures which may sometimes frame a liver cell in a benzene ring-type configuration. They open at the periphery of the lobule into the bile ducts lying in the periportal connective tissue. These bile ducts are lined by cubical epithelium. The largest of these have some smooth muscle in their walls.

The extrahepatic biliary apparatus
This consists of the right and left hepatic ducts, the gall bladder, the cystic duct and the common bile duct.

The extrahepatic ducts are lined by tall columnar epithelium. Their mucosa is highly folded and some oblique or circular smooth muscle is present in the connective tissue outside this.

The gall bladder
This organ is lined by a highly-folded mucous membrane composed of a simple columnar epithelium with a striated border, and an underlying corium of areolar tissue. No muscularis mucosae is found. The rest of the wall is of dense connective tissue containing some circular smooth muscle.

THE PANCREAS

The pancreas is an exocrine salivary gland embedded within which are endocrine portions known as the islets of Langerhans.

The exocrine pancreas
This consists of serous acini of typical form and appearance. The cells are truncated pyramids whose infra-nuclear cytoplasm is intensely basophilic and whose apical cytoplasm contains large eosinophilic zymogen granules. No myoepithelial cells are found. The centre of the acinus contains the centro-acinar cells, being the cubical lining cells of the intercalated duct which is invaginated into the acinus in the instance of the pancreas. Intralobular ducts are very rare in the pancreas. They have a lining of low columnar epithelium. Interlobular ducts lined by tall columnar epithelium run in the connective tissue septa of the gland and join up to form the main and accessory ducts which open into the duodenum.

The endocrine pancreas
There are about one million islets of Langerhans. These are clusters of epithelial cells and capillaries. The epithelial cells are of several types, but this is not manifest in sections stained by H & E. Three cell types can be made out in Azan-stained preparations. The alpha cells have red granules in their cytoplasm and tend to be arranged peripherally in the islet. They produce glucagon. The beta cells are more numerous than the alpha cells, and are more central in position. They produce insulin. They have brownish orange granules in their cytoplasm. The delta cells have small blue granules in their cytoplasm and they too lie at the periphery of the islet. Their function is unknown.

238 *Tooth (H & E)* The teeth are composed of a crown (A) and a root (B). The neck of the tooth lies at the junction of the two. The crown is composed of dentine covered by enamel and the root of dentine covered by cementum.

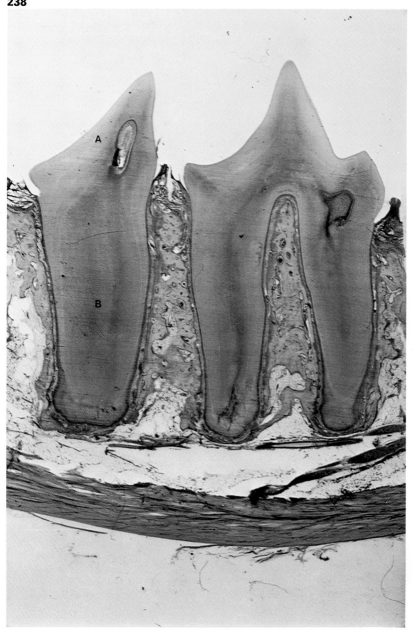

239 *Tooth (H & E)* High power of **238** to show the alveolar bone (A), periodontal membrane (B), cementum (C), and dentine (D).

240 *Tooth (Silver)* Cementum may be acellular or, as here, cellular. The cells in cellular cementum are akin to osteocytes and of stellate outline.

241 *Tooth (H & E)* High power of **239** to show compact bone of alveolus (A), periodontal membrane (B), acellular cementum (C), and dentine (D).

242 *Tooth, dentine (Silver)* High power of dentine showing tubules sectioned longitudinally. An interglobular space is arrowed.

243 *Tooth, dentine (Silver)* High power of dentine showing tubules sectioned transversely and containing odontoblast cytoplasmic processes.

239

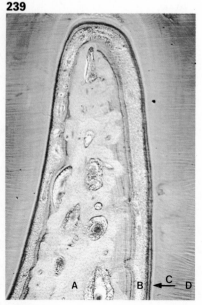

240

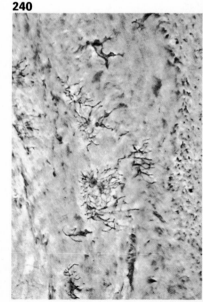

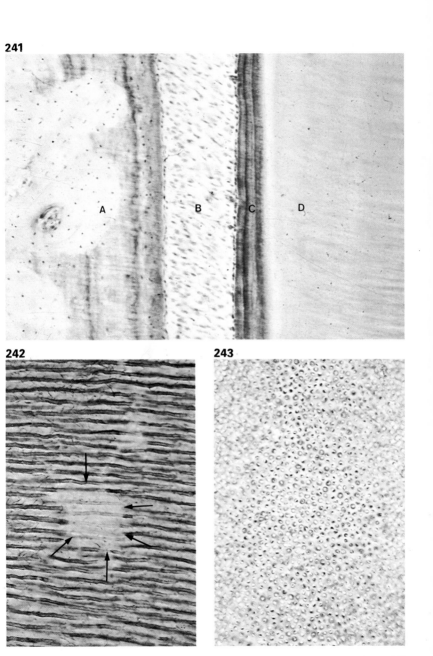

155

244 *Tooth, dentine (Silver)* High power of dentine showing a richly branching network of cytoplasmic processes derived from odontoblasts.

245 *Tooth, dentine (Silver)* Odontoblasts (A), pre-dentine (B), and dentine (C) are here shown at high power.

246 *Parotid gland (H & E)* This gland is of pure serous type. Intralobular ducts (*arrows*) are common, in striking contrast to the pancreas (which is also a salivary gland of pure serous type) in which they are relatively uncommon. An interlobular duct is seen at A.

247 *Parotid gland (H & E)* The acini of the gland (*arrows*) are purely serous. An intercalated duct (A) and an intralobular duct (B) are also present.

248 *Parotid duct (H & E)* The parotid duct is lined by stratified columnar epithelium.

244

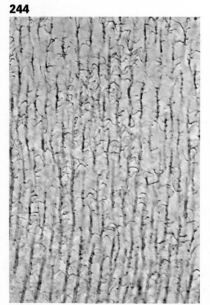

245

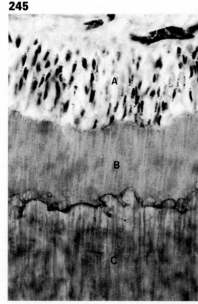

246

247

248

249 *Submandibular salivary gland (H & Alcian blue)* This gland exhibits serous (A) and mixed acini (B). An intralobular duct lies at C.

250 *Submandibular salivary gland (H & Alcian blue)* High power of **249** to show mucous acini (A) with serous crescents (B), and serous acini (C). Mucus stains blue with alcian blue. An intralobular duct (D) is also present.

251 *Submandibular salivary gland (H & E)* In the absence of special staining methods, the distinction between serous and mixed acini is difficult to draw. An intercalated duct lies at A and an intralobular duct at B.

252 *Submandibular salivary gland (H & E)* At high power, the majority of the acini in the upper part of the field are seen to be serous and those in the lower half of the frame are mainly mixed. An intercalated duct lies at A.

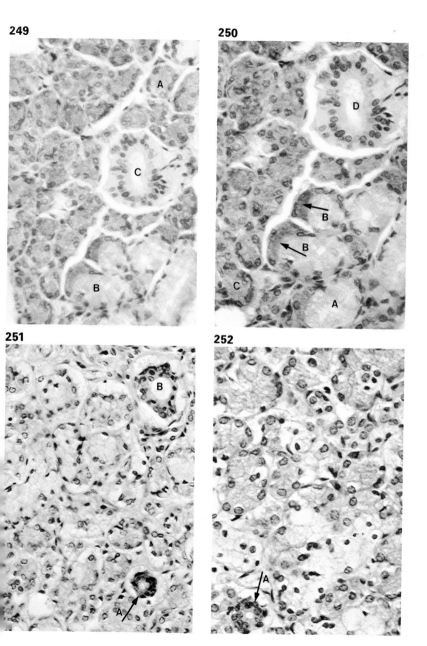

159

253 *Sublingual gland (H & E)* This is a salivary gland exhibiting mucous acini, serous acini and mixed acini.

254 *Sublingual salivary gland (Azan)* An interlobular duct lies at A and an intralobular duct at B.

255 *Sublingual salivary gland (H & E)* High power of **253** to show mucous acini (A), mixed acini (B), and serous acini (C). An intralobular (D) and an interlobular duct (E) are also seen.

256 *Sublingual salivary gland (Azan)* At high power mucous (A), mixed (B), and serous (C), acini can be seen. Intralobular (D) and interlobular (E) ducts are present.

257 *Tongue (H & E)* The tongue is covered by stratified squamous epithelium (A) resting on a corium of loose connective tissue (B). The tongue substance is composed mainly of skeletal muscle (C) with some salivary glands which are here of pure serous type (D). Filiform (E) and fungiform (F) papillae are present.

258 *Tongue (H & E)* High power of **257** to show skeletal muscle cut in LS (A) and TS (B) and pure serous glands (C).

253

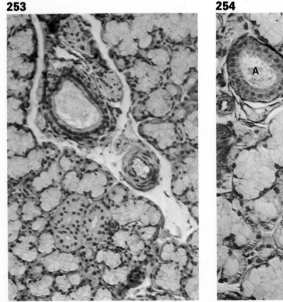

254

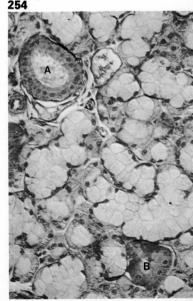

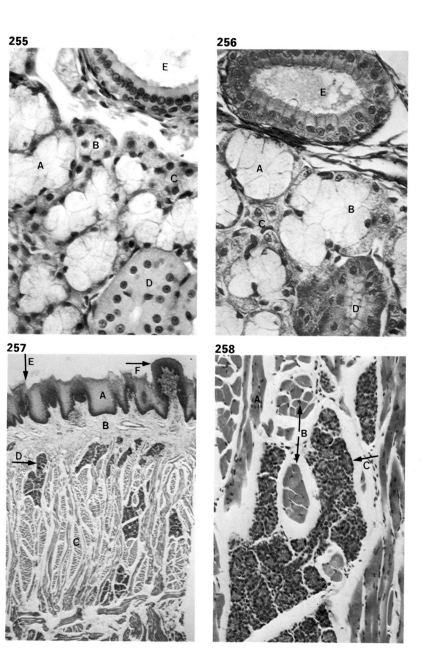

161

259 *Tongue, filiform papilla (H & E)* The papilla is a conical mass of cornified epithelial cells.

260 *Tongue, fungiform papilla (H & E)* The papilla has a core of loose connective tissue (A) and is covered by stratified squamous epithelium (B).

261 *Tongue, circumvallate papilla (H & E)* The papilla is raised only slightly above the general surface level and is surrounded by a trench (A). Taste buds (B) are present in the side walls.

262 *Tongue, glands of von Ebner (H & E)* High power of **261** to show the pure serous salivary glands associated with circumvallate papillae.

263 *Tongue, taste buds (H & OGE)* The gustatory cells (A) have oval dark nuclei and the supporting cells (B) have pale rounded nuclei. A taste pore is seen at C.

259

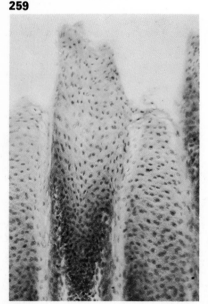

260

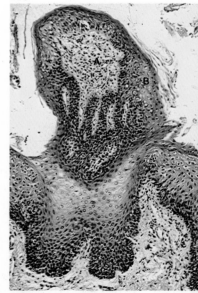

261

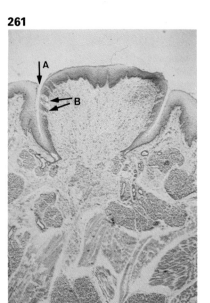

262

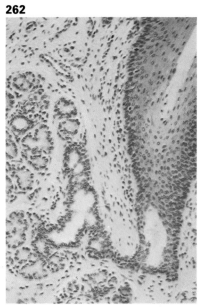

263

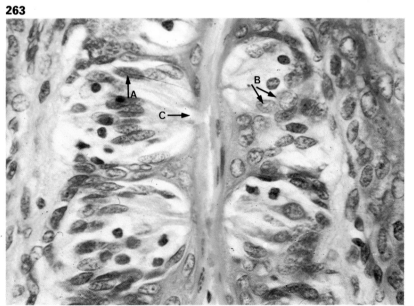

163

264 *Lip (Azan)* The lip is covered by stratified squamous epithelium of both skin (A) and mucous membrane (B) varieties. The junction of the two occurs at the red margin of the lip and the height of the epithelium increases abruptly. Hair follicles and sebaceous glands lie in the skin (C).

265 *Lip (H & E)* The main bulk of the lip is formed by the skeletal muscle of the orbicularis oris (A). Sweat glands (B) and mucous salivary glands (C) are also present.

266 *Lip (H & E)* High power of a field from **265** to show a hair follicle (A) and its associated sebaceous glands (B).

267 *Lip (H & E)* High power of **265** to show the epithelium of the muco-cutaneous junction.

264

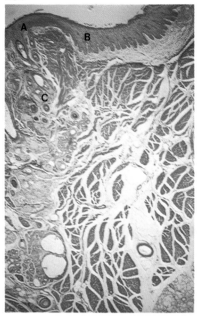

265

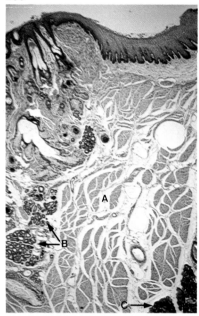

266

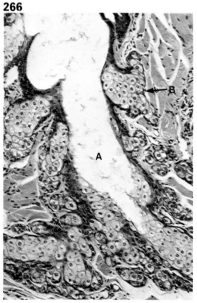

267

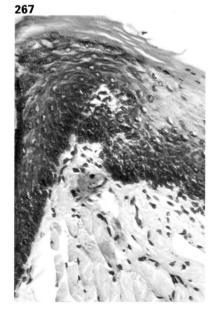

268 *Soft palate (H & E)* The soft palate is covered over most of its extent by stratified squamous epithelium of the mucous membrane variety (A). The core is of connective tissue containing solitary lymph nodules (B), skeletal muscle (C) and mucous salivary glands (D).

269 *Soft palate (H & E)* High power to show stratified squamous epithelium (A) and mucous salivary glands (B).

270 *Soft palate (H & E)* High power to show pseudo-stratified ciliated columnar epithelium (A), with a taste bud (B), mucous salivary glands (C) and their duct (D).

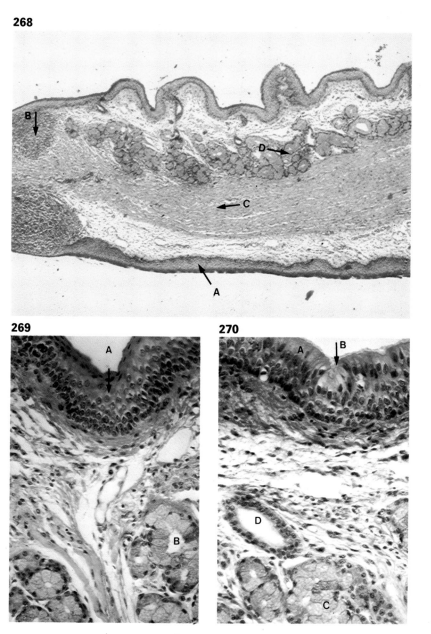

268

269

270

271 *Palatine tonsil (H & OGE)* The tonsils are masses of lymphoid tissue (A) covered by stratified squamous epithelium (B). The lymphoid tissue may be diffuse (C) or nodular (D). Mucous salivary glands are also found (E). A tonsillar crypt lies at F.

272 *Palatine tonsil (H & OGE)* High power of **271** to show the mucous acini of the tonsil.

273 *Palatine tonsil (H & E)* The stratified squamous epithelium overlying the tonsillar lymphoid tissue is often so heavily infiltrated with lymphocytes (*arrows*) as to be unrecognisable.

271

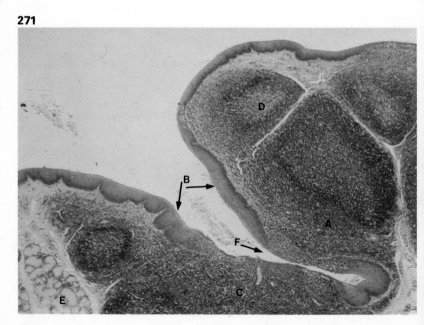

272

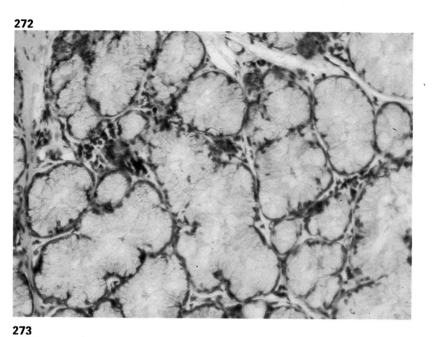

273

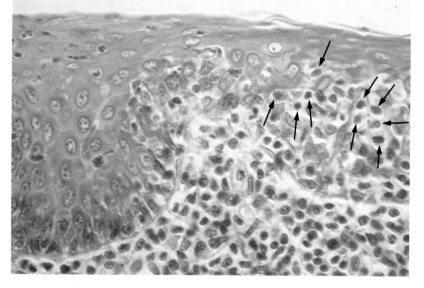

274 *TS oesophagus (H & E)* The layers of the oesophagus are:

MUCOSA   A, stratified squamous epithelium

                B, corium of loose connective tissue

                C, muscularis mucosae (smooth)

SUBMUCOSA   D, of connective tissue

MUSCULARIS   E, inner circular

                F, outer longitudinal

FIBROUS COAT   G

275 *LS oesophagus (H & OGE)* The layers are lettered as for **274**.

276 *Oesophagus (H & E)* High power of **274** to show the mucosa and part of the submucosa. The stratified squamous epithelium lies at A. The muscularis mucosae (B) is composed of longitudinally-running smooth muscle.

277 *Oesophagus (H & E)* At its upper and lower extremities, and opposite the tracheal bifurcation, the oesophagus has mucous glands in the sub-mucosa.

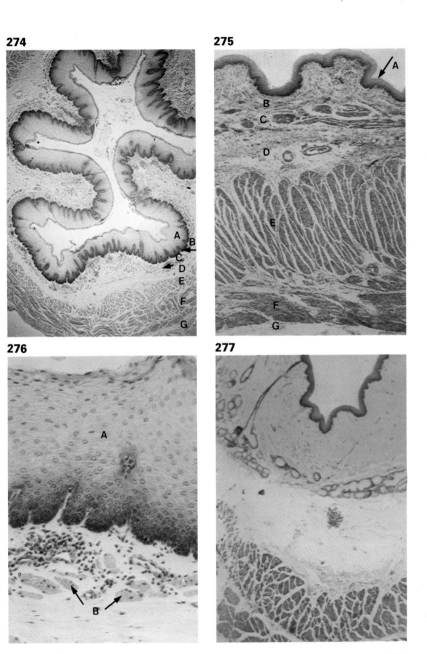

278 *Oesophagus (H & E)* Part of the inner circular (A) and part of the outer longitudinal (B) muscle coat with the plexus of Auerbach (C) between.

279 *Oesophagus (H & E)* High power of **278** to show the ganglion cells of the plexus of Auerbach.

280 *Oesophageo-cardiac junction (H & E)* The oesophagus lies to the left and the stomach to the right. The gastric pits are seen (A). There is no sphincter at the junction in the respect that the inner circular muscle coat is not thickened.

281 *Oesophageo-cardiac junction (H & E)* High power of **280** to show the abrupt change (*arrow*) between stratified squamous (*right*) and simple columnar epithelium (*left*).

278

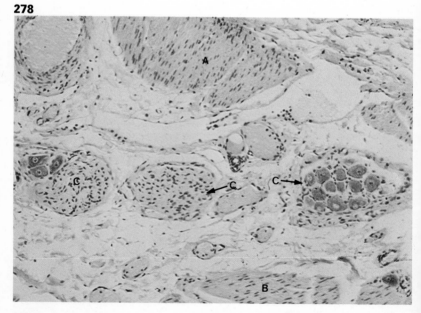

279

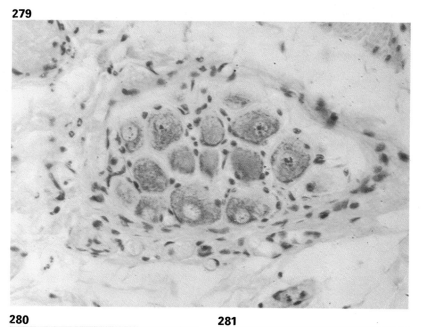

280

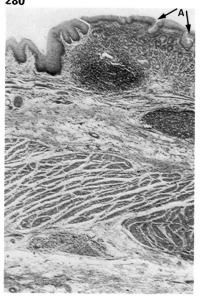

281

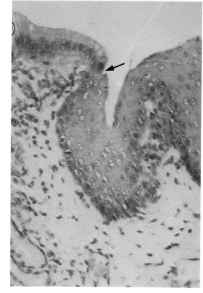

282 *Oesophageo-cardiac junction (H & PAS)* Preparation from a small rodent in which the cardiac glands stand out (*arrows*) because their content of mucus has been stained bright pink.

283 *Cardia of stomach (H & PAS)* High power of **282** to show the mucus-secreting glands found in this part of the stomach.

284 *Body of stomach (H & E)* A well-developed fold, or ruga, of the gastric mucosa is seen at A. The submucosa (B) and muscularis externa (C) are also seen.

285 *Body of stomach (H & E)* Higher power view of **284** to show the mucosa (A), submucosa (B), inner circular smooth muscle coat (C), outer longitudinal smooth muscle coat (D), and serous coat (E).

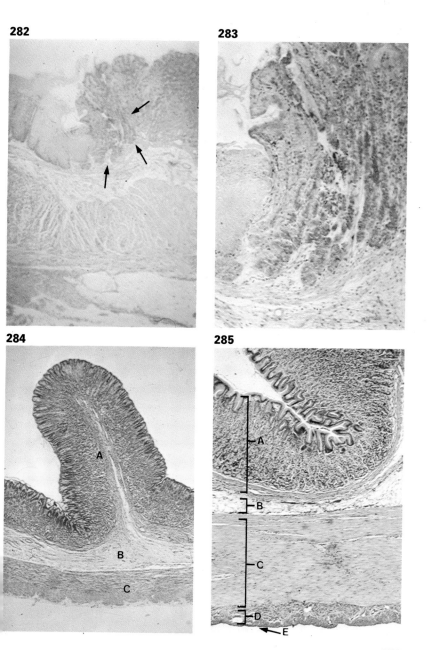

282

283

284

285

286 *Body of stomach (H & E)* The mucosa or mucous membrane of the stomach lies in this field. It is composed of a lining of simple columnar epithelium (A) which dips in to form the gastric pits (B) into which open th simple test-tube glands (C) of the body.

287 *Body of stomach (H & E)* High power of **286** to show the gastric pits (A) and the neck region of the fundic glands (B). Oxyntic cells (C) are mor common in the neck than in the deeper part of the gland.

288 *Body of stomach (H & E)* High power of **286** to show the deep part of the fundic glands. The peptic cells (A) are pale and more common in this part of the gland. The oxyntic cells (B) are strongly eosinophilic.

289 *Body of stomach (H & E)* A fundic gland (A) is cut longitudinally. It is lined by peptic cells (B) and oxyntic cells (C).

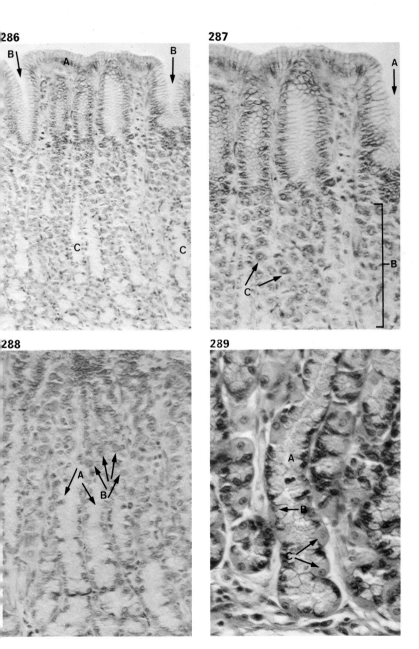

290 *Body of stomach (H & E)* Fundic glands are here sectioned transversely. The pale peptic cells (A) lie next to the lumen. The oxyntic cells (B) are eosinophilic and lie against the basement membrane.

291 *Pylorus of stomach (H & OGE)* The gastric pits (A) are deeper in the pylorus than in the body. The pyloric glands (B) are simple test-tubes and secrete mucus. The inner circular muscle coat is greatly thickened to form the pyloric sphincter (C).

292 *Pylorus of stomach (H & OGE)* High power of **291** to show the mucosa of the pylorus. The gastric pits (A) are deep. The pyloric glands (B) are simple tubular and mucus-secreting.

290

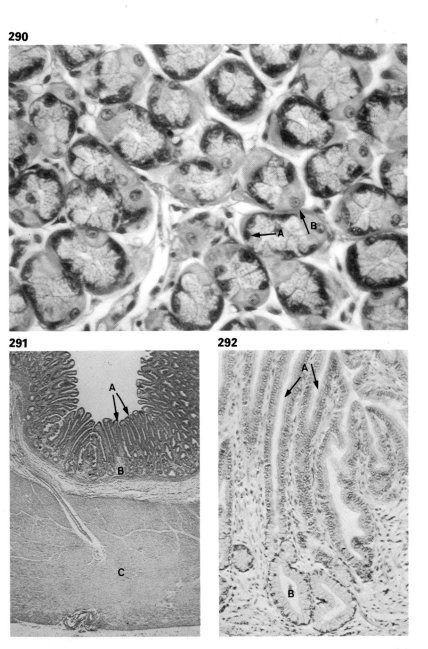

291

292

293 *Pyloro-duodenal junction (Azan)* The pylorus lies on the right and the duodenum on the left. The thickening of the inner circular muscle coat to form the pyloric sphincter is seen at A. The mucosal change from gastric pits (B) to small intestinal villi (C) takes place at D. Several solitary lymphoid nodules are also present (E).

294 *Small intestine (Azan)* The four layers common to most parts of the alimentary canal are here present. They are the mucosa (A), submucosa (B), muscularis (C) and serosa (D). The mucosa is thrown into villous folds (E). The lining epithelium dips in to form the crypts of Lieberkühn (F).

295 *Small intestine, plica connivens (H & E)* The plicae conniventes are folds of mucosa (A) and submucosa (B) combined. They are most prevalent in the terminal duodenum and upper jejunum, and are absent entirely in the terminal ileum.

293

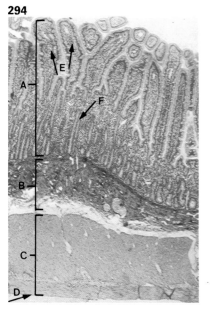

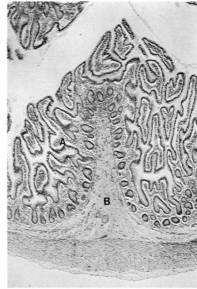

296 *Small intestine, villus (H & E)* The villi are covered by columnar epithelium with a striated border and containing scattered goblet cells. The core of the villus is the loose connective tissue of the lamina propria and contains smooth muscle bundles (*arrows*) derived from the muscularis mucosae.

297 *Small intestine, villi (H & E)* The central lacteal is well demonstrated in each of the three villi shown. It is a lymphatic capillary lined by endothelium.

298 *Small intestine, crypts of Lieberkühn (H & E)* The crypts are test-tube shaped invaginations of the lining epithelium. Mitotic figures (*arrowed*) are common in the epithelial cells of the crypts.

299 *Small intestine, crypts of Lieberkühn (H & E)* The crypts are coiled and are often seen cut transversely, as here. Again note the high number of mitotic figures in the epithelium (*arrows*).

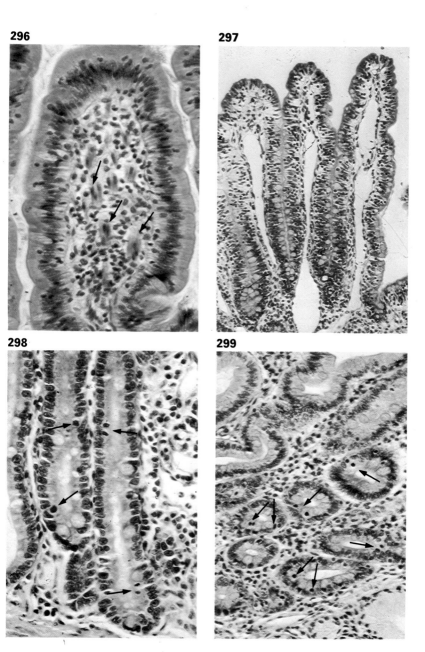

296

297

298

299

300 *Small intestine, Paneth cells (Dithizone)* In this longitudinally-sectioned crypt the Paneth cells are seen to lie at the base of the crypt (*arrows*). Their supranuclear granules have stained brown.

301 *Small intestine, Paneth cells (Dithizone)* The Paneth cells (*arrows*) are clearly seen in these transverse profiles of crypts near their bases.

302 *Small intestine, submucosa (H & E)* The submucosa is mainly collagenous with fibroblast cells whose nuclei can be seen throughout the field. A portion of the plexus of Meissner can be seen in the upper part of the field (*arrows*).

303 *Small intestine, muscularis externa (H & E)* The muscle coat of the gut is arranged in inner circular (*top*) and outer longitudinal (*bottom*) layers of smooth muscle.

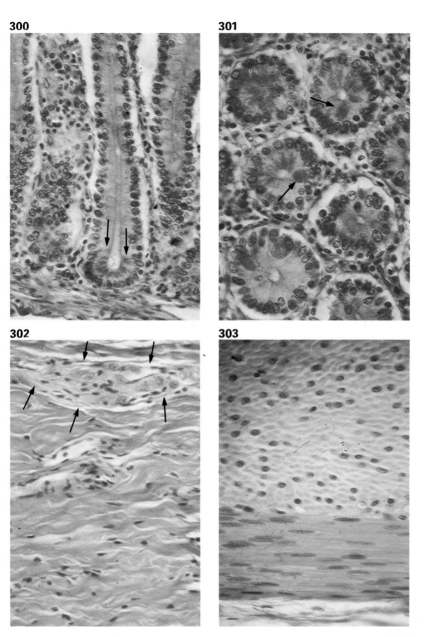

304 *Duodenum (H & E)* The duodenum differs from the other parts of the small gut in the respect that the glands of Brunner (*arrows*) lie in the submucosa.

305 *Duodenum, Brunner's glands (H & E)* Under high power the glands are seen to contain only one type of cell. The glands are mucus-secreting.

306 *Ileum, Peyer's patch (H & E)* The Peyer's patches are confined to the antimesenteric border of the ileum and are aggregations of lymphoid tissue in the lamina propria. Over the patches villi are present in reduced numbers.

307 *Ileum, Peyer's patch (H & E)* Medium power of **306** to show two lymphoid nodules (A). The submucosa lies at B and the muscularis at C.

308 *Ileum, Peyer's patch (H & E)* High power of **306** to show the lymphoid mass.

304

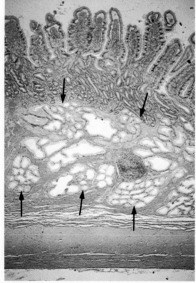

305

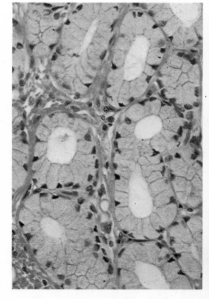

306

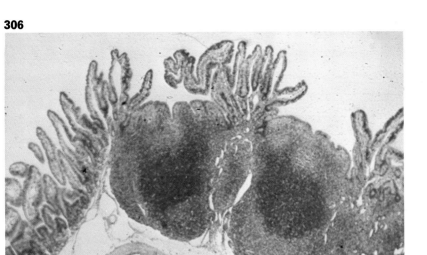

307

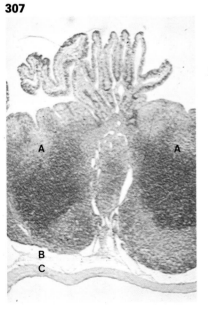

308

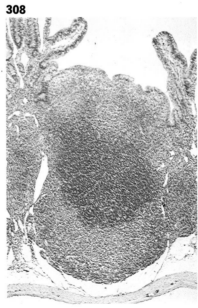

187

309 *Large intestine (H & E)* The large gut differs from the small in the respect that villi are lacking, and hence crypts alone are found in the mucosa. The outer longitudinal coat of smooth muscle is present in the form of three disconnected bands (taeniae) one of which lies in the plane of section of this preparation.

310 *Large intestine (H & E)* High power of **309** to show the crypts of the large gut. They are lined by an epithelium similar to that lining those of the small gut, i.e. simple columnar with striated border, but goblet cells are here more numerous.

311 *Vermiform appendix (H & E)* The appendix in general has the same structure as the large intestine. It has lymphoid tissue in the mucosa around its complete circumference and has a complete outer longitudinal muscle coat.

312 *Vermiform appendix (H & E)* High power of **311** to show the massive lymphocytic infiltration in the mucosa. The lining epithelium is simple columnar.

309

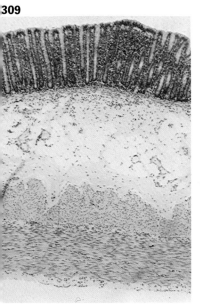

310

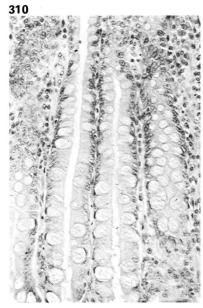

311

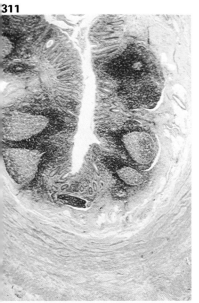

312

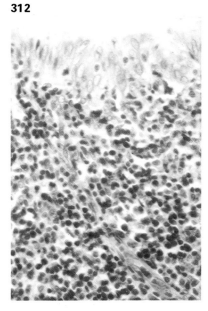

313 *Anal canal (H & E)* This longitudinal section of the anal canal in a small rodent shows that the viscus has a different morphology in each of its upper (A), middle (B), and lower (C) thirds.

314 *Anal canal (H & E)* Higher power view of area A from **313**. The anal canal in its upper third has the same structure as the large intestine.

315 *Anal canal (H & E)* Higher power view of area B from **313**. In the intermediate third the anal canal is lined by stratified squamous epithelium of mucous membrane type (A). The smooth muscle of the internal (involuntary) sphincter lies at B. Sweat glands (C) of modified type are also present.

313

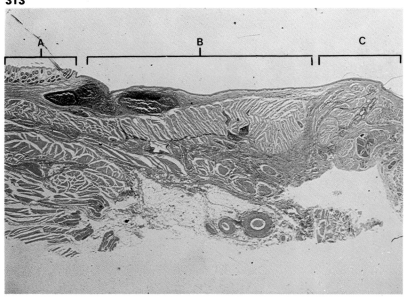

A   B   C

314

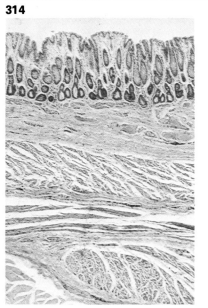

315

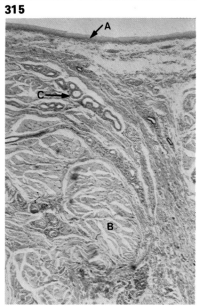

A

C

B

316 *Anal canal (H & E)* High power of **315** to show the modified sweat glands found in the anal region. The glands are lined by a simple cubical epithelium and have a large lumen. They resemble the 'apocrine' glands of the skin.

317 *Anal canal (H & E)* High power of area C from **313**. The terminal part of the anal canal is lined by skin (A) containing hair follicles with sebaceous glands (B). Circum-anal or hepatoid glands also occur (C). Skeletal muscle of the external (voluntary) sphincter is present (D).

318 *Anal canal (H & E)* High power of a field from **317** to show typical sebaceous glands (A) clustered around a hair follicle (B).

319 *Anal canal (H & E)* High power of **317** to show circum-anal (hepatoid) glands (A) opening by means of a duct (B) into a hair follicle (C). Sebaceous glands are also present (D).

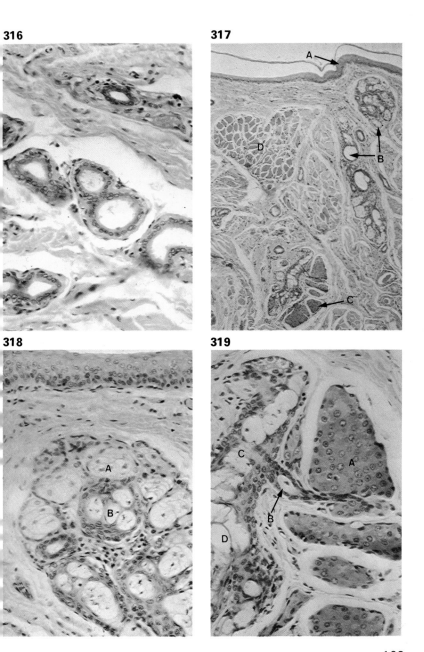

193

320 *Liver (H & E)* The liver lobules are well-defined in some animals such as the pig because the periportal connective tissue is extensively developed.

321 *Liver (H & E)* A lobule from human liver. A central vein lies near the centre of the field and the periportal connective tissue lies at the bottom of the field.

322 *Liver (H & E)* High power of the central vein from **321**. It is lined by endothelium and has hepatic sinusoids entering all round.

323 *Liver (Azan)* A central vein (A) into which liver sinusoids (B) are discharging is shown here. The central vein is partly filled with blood (C).

324 *Liver (H & E)* Periportal connective tissue (A), containing branches of the hepatic artery (B), and portal vein (C), and a bile duct (D) and a lymphatic (E).

325 *Liver (Alkaline phosphatase)* The bile canaliculi are rich in the enzyme alkaline phosphatase and by applying the histochemical reaction for this enzyme to liver tissue, the bile canaliculi are outlined by deposits of cobalt sulphide, which is black.

320

321

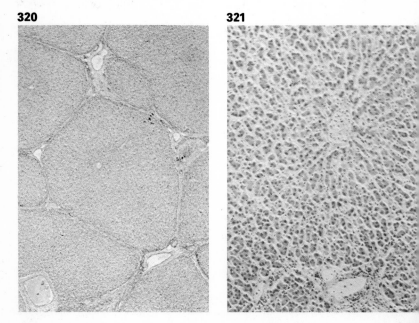

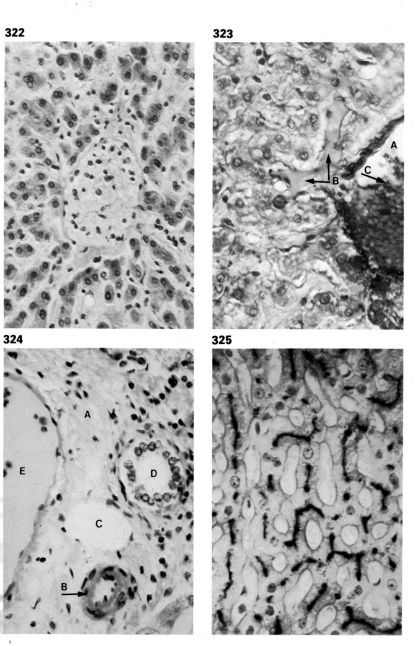

322

323

A

B

C

324

A

E

D

C

B

325

195

326 *Liver (H & E)* Indian ink administered intravenously is phagocytosed as here, by the macrophages lining the hepatic sinusoids (*arrows*).

327 *Liver (PAS & Silver & H)* The reticular fibre framework of the liver is revealed by silver impregnation. The fibres (*arrows*) frame the liver sinusoids.

328 *Gall bladder (H & E)* The gall bladder has a mucosa which is highly folded (A), a fibrous submucosa (B), a smooth muscle coat (C) and a fibrous adventitia (D).

329 *Gall bladder (H & E)* High power of **328** to show a mucosal fold. The lining epithelium is simple columnar with a striated border.

330 *Gall bladder (H & E)* High power of **328** to show the submucosa (A), smooth muscle coat (B), and fibrous adventitia (C), covered by serosal endothelium (D).

326
327

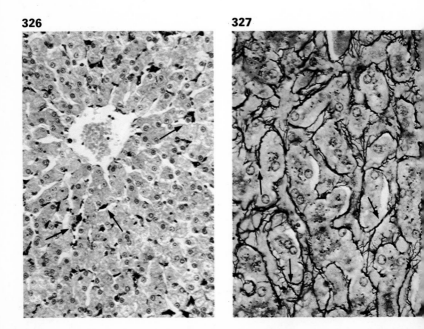

328

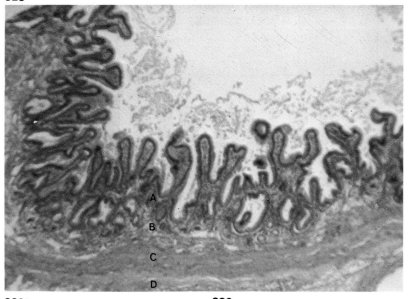

A

B

C

D

329

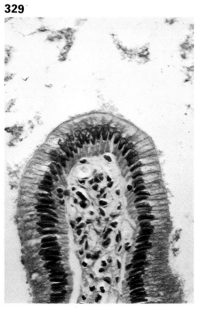

330

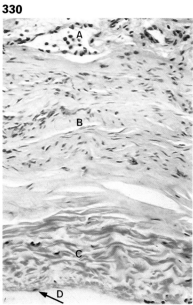

A

B

C

D

331 *Pancreas (Gomori's Chrome-alum/H)* The exocrine part of the gland is composed of serous acini (A). Intralobular ducts are rare in the pancreas. An interlobular duct lies at B. The endocrine portion of the pancreas consists of the islets of Langerhans (C).

332 *Pancreas (H & E)* High power to show an islet of Langerhans (A) and an interlobular duct (B) surrounded by serous acini.

333 *Pancreas (H & E)* High power to show serous acini with peripheral basophilia (A) and centro-acinar cell nuclei (B). An intercalated duct lies at C.

334 *Pancreas (H & E)* The main duct of the pancreas is illustrated here. It is lined by columnar epithelium with goblet cells and is surrounded by dense connective tissue.

331

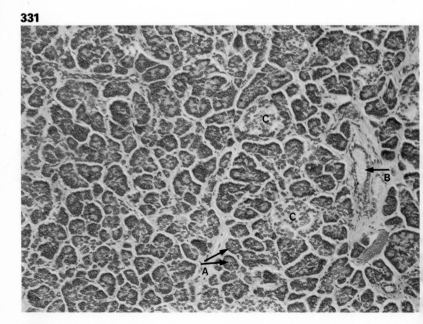

332

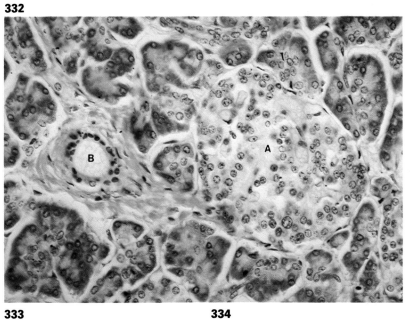

333

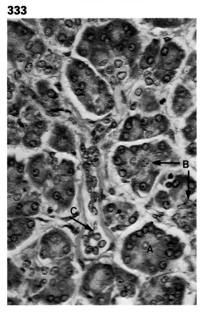

334

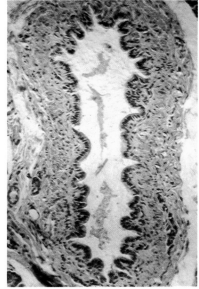

335 *Pancreas (Gomori's Chrome-alum/H)* Two islets of Langerhans lie in this field and their high vascularity is reflected in the large numbers of capillaries present (*arrows*).

336 *Pancreas (Azan)* The upper right segment of the field is occupied by an islet in which the alpha and beta cells are now stained pink and purple respectively.

337 *Pancreas (Gomori)* An islet showing alpha cells stained pink and beta cells stained blue.

335

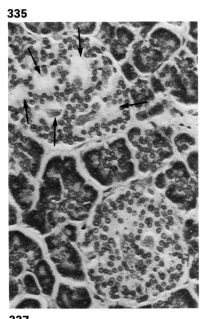

336

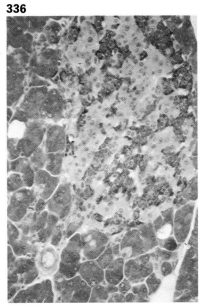

337

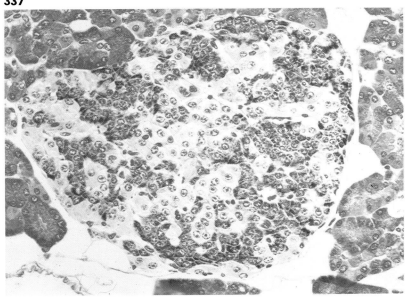

The Respiratory System

THE NOSE AND LARYNX

The mucous membrane of the upper respiratory tract (i.e. of nasal cavity, paranasal air sinuses, larynx, trachea and bronchi) is composed of pseudo-stratified ciliated columnar epithelium resting on a highly vascular corium. Goblet cells are found in the epithelium. The corium is densely adherent to the underlying hyaline cartilage or bone which keeps the tract patent. The corium also contains mucous and serous glands. Muscle is also found, and may be smooth or skeletal.

The nose
The front of the vestibule is lined by epidermis with coarse hairs and sebaceous glands. The back of the vestibule is covered by a mucous membrane covered with stratified squamous epithelium of the mucous membrane variety.

The remainder of the nasal cavity is lined by pseudo-stratified ciliated columnar epithelium with goblet cells. The cilia beat towards the pharynx. The corium is very vascular and warms the inspired air. It contains mixed salivary glands. Outside the corium is hyaline cartilage or compact bone.

The epiglottis
This is covered on its superior aspect and for most of its inferior aspect by stratified squamous epithelium of the mucous membrane variety; this gives way to stratified columnar epithelium and then to pseudo-stratified ciliated columnar epithelium with goblet cells. Taste buds are found in the stratified columnar epithelium. The epithelio-corial junction is scalloped on the lingual aspect and plane on the laryngeal side. The core is of elastic cartilage which has several perforations. Mixed salivary glands are also found in the corium, especially on the laryngeal aspect.

The larynx
This is lined everywhere by pseudo-stratified ciliated columnar epithelium except for the vocal folds, which are covered by stratified squamous epithelium of the mucous membrane variety. Cartilage and skeletal muscle lie everywhere in the wall. The cartilage is hyaline throughout except for the corniculate, cuneiform and the vocal process of the arytenoid cartilage, which are elastic. Mixed salivary glands lie in the wall.

THE TRACHEA AND LUNG

The trachea and extrapulmonary bronchi
These have an identical structure. The inner lining is of pseudo-stratified ciliated columnar epithelium with some goblet cells. This rests on a corium of loose connective tissue containing many longitudinally-running elastic fibres. Mixed

salivary glands opening into the lumen by short ducts lie in the corium. Outside the corium is a ∩-shaped piece of hyaline cartilage with the gap on the posterior aspect. Smooth muscle fibres bridge the interval between the ends of the cartilage. On the outside is a fibrous coat.

The lung

The lung is a compound tubulo-alveolar gland. The alveoli of the lung correspond to the secretory segment of such a gland and the bronchioles, bronchi and trachea are comparable with a system of ducts. The lung is covered on its surface by highly elastic loose connective tissue covered by endothelium; together these constitute the visceral pleura. Septa of connective tissue pass into the lung substance from the hilum dividing it into lobules. Intrapulmonary bronchi have the same structure as the extrapulmonary bronchi with the exception that the smooth muscle is distributed all round the wall in spiral fashion and the cartilage is arranged in irregular plaques. The basic unit of lung tissue is a bronchiole and its subsequent subdivisions, of alveolar duct, alveolar sac and alveoli.

Bronchioles are bronchi lacking cilia, glands and cartilage. Their wall is composed therefore of a lining of simple low columnar or cubical epithelium resting on a highly elastic corium. Outside this is a complete cuff of smooth muscle. Respiratory bronchioles are bronchioles studded at intervals along one side with alveoli lined by pavement epithelium; a branch of the pulmonary artery runs along the other side of the respiratory bronchiole.

The alveolar duct is comparable to a long passage flanked by pillars on either side. The pillars have the same structure as bronchioles. Between the pillars lie the alveolar sacs which have no wall since they are the central passage into which many alveoli open.

The pulmonary alveoli are lined by extremely attenuated epithelial cells with here and there a cubical cell. Outside the epithelium is a film of connective tissue composed of reticular and elastic fibres and supporting an enormous capillary bed. Free macrophages (dust cells) lie on the surface of the epithelium.

338 *Epiglottis (Weigert's elastic)* The epiglottic cartilage is elastic in type, and is perforated as at A. Salivary glands of mixed type (B) lie in or near the perforations. The epithelium on the superior surface is stratified squamous (C) and on the inferior, pseudo-stratified columnar (D).

339 *Epiglottis (Weigert's elastic)* High power of **338** to show the elastic cartilage. The chondrocytes (A) are embedded in a matrix rich in elastic fibres.

340 *Epiglottis (Weigert's elastic)* High power of **338** to show the salivary glands. They are mucous in type with serous crescents. A duct lined with cubical epithelium lies at A.

341 *Epiglottis (Weigert's elastic)* High power of **338** to show the stratified squamous epithelium covering the upper surface of the epiglottis.

338

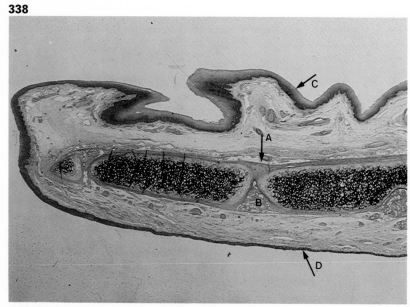

339

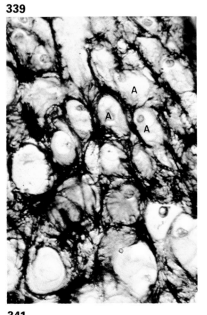

340

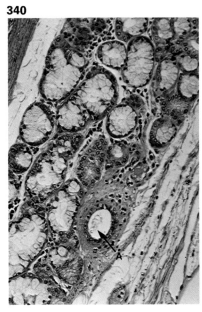

341

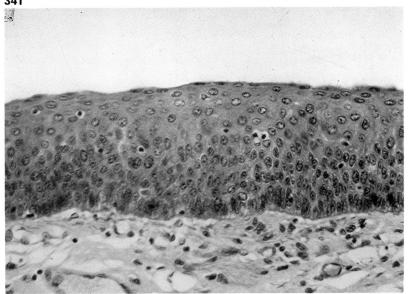

342 *Epiglottis (Weigert's elastic)* High power of **338** to show the stratified ciliated columnar epithelium on the inferior aspect of the epiglottis. Two taste buds are present (*arrows*).

343 *Larynx (H & E)* The thyroid (A), cricoid (B), and arytenoid (C) cartilages have been sectioned. The lining epithelium is ciliated columnar except over the vocal processes (D), where it is stratified squamous. Mixed glands lie at E. The oesophagus is sectioned at F.

344 *Larynx (H & E)* High power of **343** to show the vocal process (A), arytenoid cartilage (B), cricoid cartilage (C), and mixed glands (D). The epithelial change occurs at the arrow.

345 *Nasal cavity (H & E)* This preparation from a kitten shows the septal cartilage (A), the hard palate (B), and part of the lateral wall (C). A more complex conchal pattern is present than would be the case in man.

346 *Nasal cavity (H & E)* High power of **345** to show the nasal septum. The change from ciliated columnar epithelium (*bottom*) to olfactory epithelium (*top*) occurs at the arrows. The septal cartilage (A) is hyaline.

342

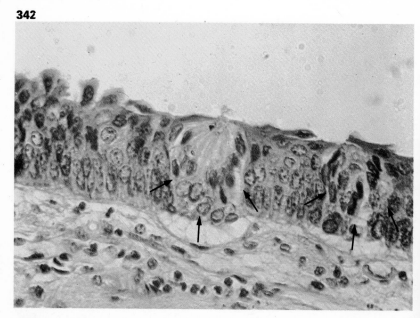

206

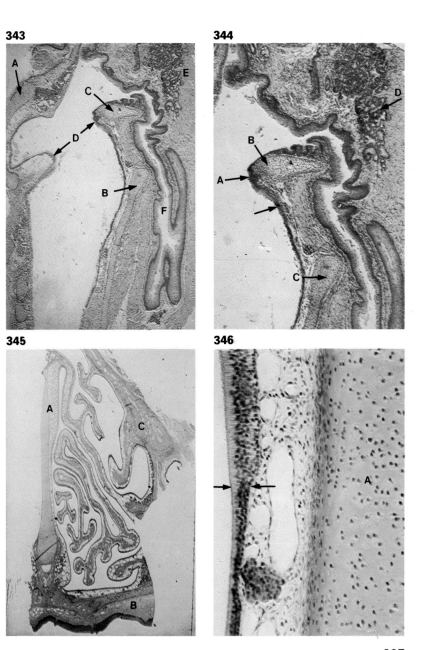

347 *Nasal cavity (H & E)* The epithelia of the nasal cavity are here shown under high power. The olfactory epithelium (*top*) is described on page 302.

348 *Nasal cavity (H & E)* High power of **345** to show the mucosa of the respiratory portion of the nasal cavity. The epithelium is ciliated columnar and rests on a highly vascular corium containing mixed salivary glands.

349 *TS trachea (H & E + Toluidin blue)* The anterior wall and parts of the side wall are shown. The hyaline cartilage is stained dark purple.

350 *LS trachea (H & E + Toluidin blue)* Three tracheal cartilages are sectioned. The cartilage is again dark purple in colour with this stain. The pulmonary artery or the aorta also lies in the field (*arrow*).

351 *TS trachea (H & OGE)* This field from the posterior wall of the trachea shows the free ends of the tracheal cartilages (A) and the smooth (trachealis) muscle (B) in the gap.

347

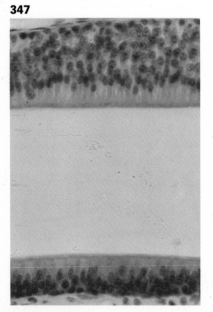

348

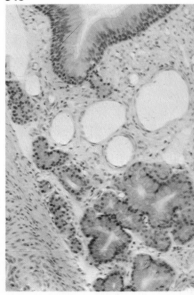

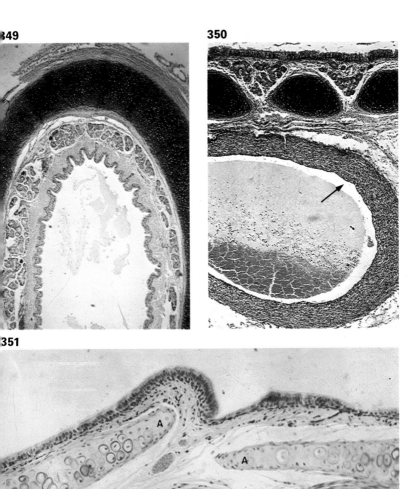

352 *TS trachea (H & E)* At medium power the lining epithelium (A), mixed salivary glands (B), hyaline cartilage (C) and fibrous corium (D) can be discerned.

353 *TS trachea (Weigert's elastic)* In this preparation the rich content of elastic fibres in the lamina propria is shown (*arrows*).

354 *LS trachea (H & E)* The columnar epithelium (A), and mixed salivary glands (B) are seen. The glands are more common between the cartilaginous rings (C). The fibrous coat lies at D.

355 *Trachea (H & E)* The pseudo-stratified ciliated columnar epithelium (A) rests on loose connective tissue (B). A mucous (C) and a serous acinus (D) are also seen.

356 *Intrapulmonary bronchus (Masson)* The goblet cells (*arrows*) in the lining epithelium are stained blue by this method.

352
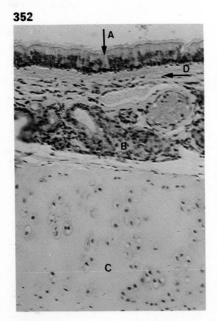

353
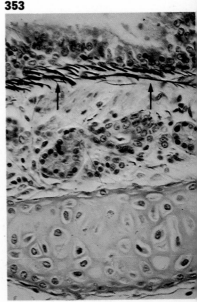

354

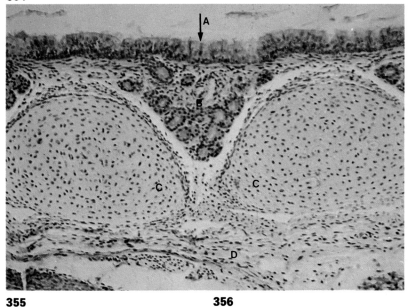

355

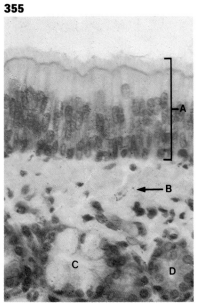

356

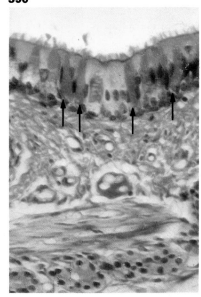

357 *Intrapulmonary bronchus (H & E + Toluidin blue)* The cartilage, here stained dark purple, in the wall of the intrapulmonary bronchus is present in the form of irregular plaques (*arrows*). Lung tissue occupies the lower two-thirds of the field.

358 *Intrapulmonary bronchus (H & E + Toluidin blue)* High power of **357** to show the lining epithelium (A), mixed salivary glands (B), smooth muscle (C) and hyaline cartilage (D).

359 *Lung (H & E + Toluidin blue)* The pleura lies at A. Small intra-pulmonary bronchi (B) and pulmonary alveoli (C) are present. A bronchiole (D) has also been sectioned. A branch of the pulmonary artery lies at E.

360 *Lung, small intrapulmonary bronchus (H & E + Toluidin blue)* High power of **359** to show an intrapulmonary bronchus. A small plaque of cartilage (A) indicates that the structure is a bronchus.

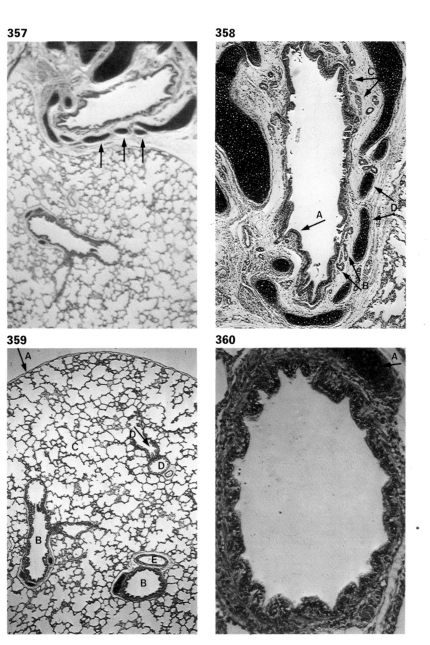

357

358

359

360

213

361 *Lung, bronchiole (H & E + Toluidin blue)* A bronchiole has been sectioned in both transverse (*bottom*) and longitudinal (*top*) directions. Cartilage and salivary glands are absent.

362 *Lung, bronchiole (Nuclear fast red)* Several free macrophages (dust cells) filled with ingested carbon lie on the surface of the bronchiolar epithelium.

363 *Lung, bronchiole (Weigert's elastic)* The rich plexus (*arrows*) of elastic fibres in the mucosa of a bronchiole is here illustrated. Two dust cells lie at A.

364 *Lung (Weigert's elastic)* High power view of pulmonary alveoli. A small blood vessel lies at A and contains several red cells and one white cell. It has a rich plexus of elastic fibres in its wall. Pulmonary alveoli with their elastic fibres are seen at B.

361

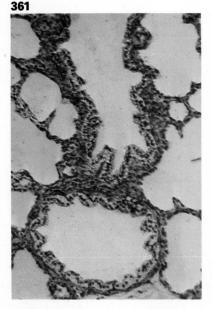

362

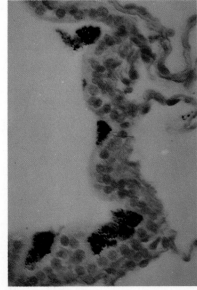

363

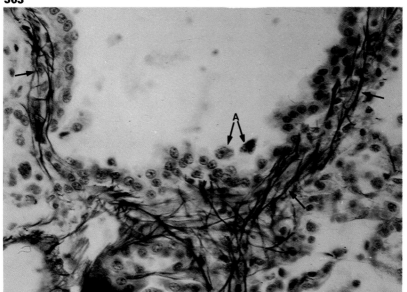

364

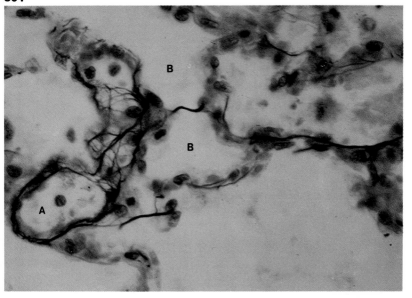

The Urinary System

THE KIDNEY

The kidney is composed of units known as pyramids, which constitute the medulla of the kidney. The renal cortex lies superficial to, and between the pyramids. The renal artery enters at the hilum and divides into several large branches which pass between the pyramids and then arch over in the boundary zone between cortex and medulla as the arciform arteries. From these, smaller arteries pass into the cortex. The arterioles derived from the cortical arteries divide into a capillary tuft (glomerulus) and the capillaries reassemble to form yet another (efferent) arteriole which emerges from the glomerulus at the same point as the ingoing (afferent) arteriole. This is the vascular pole of the glomerulus. The efferent arterioles of the superficial glomeruli break up into a capillary network to supply the other cortical structures, whilst the efferent arterioles of the juxta-medullary glomeruli pass into the medulla as the vasa recta before breaking into a network of capillaries to supply the medullary tissues. Veins at the cortico-medullary junction receive tributaries from both cortex and medulla. They are drained in turn by veins which pass between the pyramids to unite at the hilum to form the renal vein.

The functional unit of the kidney is the nephron, which consists of a glomerulus and its associated epithelial-lined uriniferous tubule. The latter commences as a blind tubule which surrounds the glomerulus everywhere except at its vascular pole and which is known as the capsule of Bowman: it possesses visceral and parietal layers of squamous epithelium with a lumen between. The visceral layer is applied closely to the surface of the glomerular capillaries. The complex of glomerulus and its capsule of Bowman is known as a renal corpuscle (of Malpighii). The lumen of the capsule of Bowman is continuous with the lumen of the next portion of the uriniferous tubule (i.e. the proximal convoluted tubule) at that pole of the renal corpuscle opposite to the vascular pole, the so-called urinary pole. The proximal convoluted tubule is lined by truncated pyramidal cells with a pronounced brush border and strongly eosinophilic cytoplasm. Following this is the loop of Henle which passes into the medulla and then returns to the cortex. The first part of the loop, or thin limb, is lined by squamous epithelium. The second part of the loop is lined by cubical epithelium and has a wide lumen: it is known as the thick limb. After the thick limb is another (the distal) convoluted tubule which lies within the cortex but which is only one third as long as the proximal convoluted tubule. The distal convoluted tubule is lined by cubical epithelium: it returns at one point to its renal corpuscle of origin where it forms, with the afferent arteriole, a complex known as the juxta-glomerular apparatus. The final portion of the nephron is the collecting tubule, which is lined by columnar epithelium. Several collecting tubules unite to form the duct of Bellini which opens at the apex of the pyramid into one of the major calyces of the kidney.

The juxta-glomerular apparatus lies at the vascular pole of the glomerulus and in it the wall of the afferent arteriole and of the distal convoluted tubule both exhibit modifications. The epithelium of the distal tubule shows a localised thickening of the lining known as the macula densa. The smooth muscle cells of the afferent arteriole are in intimate contact with the epithelial cells of the macula densa: they are known as juxta-glomerular cells and contain conspicuous granules in their cytoplasm. They are thought to produce renin.

The major and minor calyces and the pelvis of the kidney are lined by transitional epithelium.

THE URETER

The ureter is lined by transitional epithelium resting on a corium of loose connective tissue. The mucosa is usually thrown into longitudinal folds by the contraction of the ureteric muscle and the lumen is usually stellate in outline as a result. The corium blends into a submucosa of loose connective tissue which does not become folded when the muscle contracts. The muscle is smooth throughout and is disposed in a thin inner longitudinal layer, often amounting to little more than a film, and a hefty outer circular layer. Near the bladder, some longitudinal muscle is found outside the circular. The outer coat is of adipose tissue (retroperitoneal fat) containing blood vessels and nerves. No serosa is to be found.

THE BLADDER

The bladder is essentially an enlarged lower ureteric segment covered by serosa. It is lined by transitional epithelium resting on a corium of loose connective tissue and the mucosa is usually highly folded. A submucosa of loose connective tissue is found. The muscle is smooth and arranged in inner longitudinal, middle circular and outer longitudinal layers. Groups of parasympathetic ganglion cells are found between the muscle layers. A serous coat is present on the outside except for the base of the bladder.

THE URETHRA

The urethra in the female is short and is lined successively by epithelium of the transitional, stratified columnar and stratified squamous types. Outside the epithelium is some connective tissue with inner circular and outer longitudinal smooth muscle outside this.

The male urethra serves a dual purpose as the terminal duct of both the urinary and genital systems. It will be described in the next chapter.

365 *Kidney (Azan)* The cortex lies superficial to (A), and extends between (B) the medullary pyramids (C). An arciform artery (D) lies at the cortico-medullary junction.

366 *Renal cortex (H & E)* Three glomeruli lie in the field (*arrows*). They are surrounded by convoluted tubules of proximal and distal type.

367 *Renal cortex (H & E)* Cross sectional profiles of proximal (A) and distal (B) convoluted tubules. The proximal tubules are more eosinophilic, have a smaller lumen and taller cells than the distal convoluted tubules.

368 *Renal cortex (H & E)* Longitudinal sections of proximal (A) and distal (B) convoluted tubules are illustrated. Part of a glomerulus lies at C.

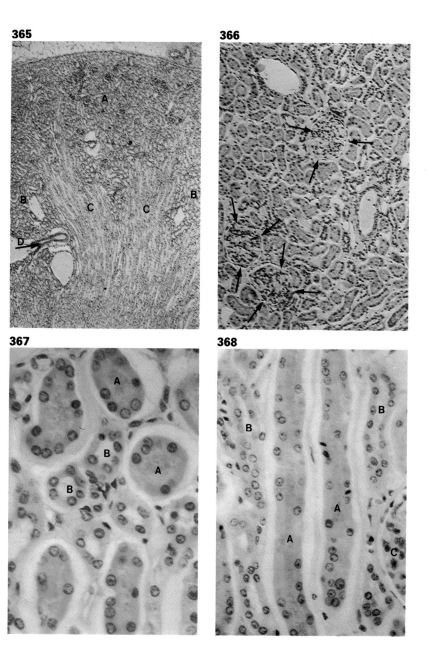

369 *Renal cortex (H & E)* A glomerulus (A), proximal convoluted tubules (B) and a distal convoluted tubule (C) occupy the field. The vascular pole of the glomerulus lies at D and the macula densa of the distal tubule at E.

370 *Renal cortex (H & E)* A glomerulus (A) with its urinary pole (B) where the lumen of the capsule of Bowman is in continuity with that of the proximal convoluted tubule (C) are the features of this field.

371 *Renal medulla (H & E)* This field is from the subcortical zone and shows proximal convoluted tubules (A), thick limbs of the loop of Henle (B), and a collecting duct (C).

369

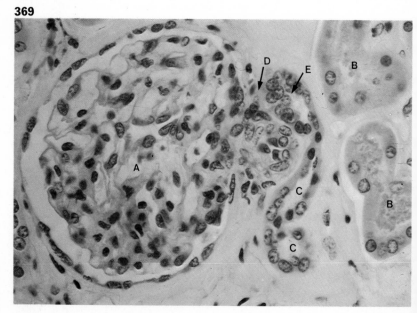

370

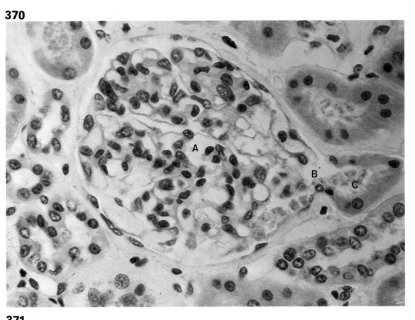

371

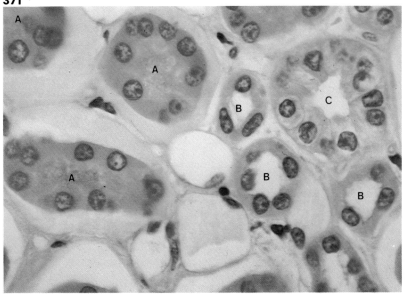

221

372 *Renal medulla (H & E)* This field from the outer medulla shows thin and thick limbs of the loop of Henle and a collecting duct (A).

373 *Renal medulla (H & E)* High power of **372** to show thick limbs (A) of the loop of Henle. The structures labelled B may be either blood vessels or thin limbs of the loop of Henle.

374 *Ureter (Van Gieson)* The lining epithelium (A) is transitional. The fibrous lamina propria (B) is stained orange-red. The muscularis (C) is of smooth muscle.

375 *Ureter (Van Gieson)* High power of **374**. The muscularis is arranged in inner circular (A) and outer longitudinal (B) layers of smooth muscle.

376 *Ureter (H & E)* The ureteric lumen is stellate. The corium and muscularis are both stained pink and are not differentiated by this stain. The outer adventitia contains the ureteric blood vessels (*arrows*).

377 *Ureter (H & E)* High power of **376** to show the transitional epithelium (A), and longitudinal (B), circular (C), and longitudinal (D) layers of smooth muscle.

372

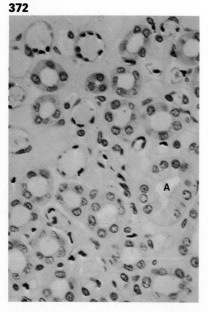

373

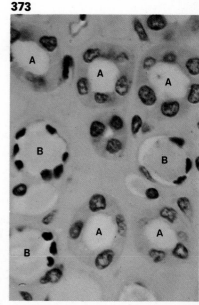

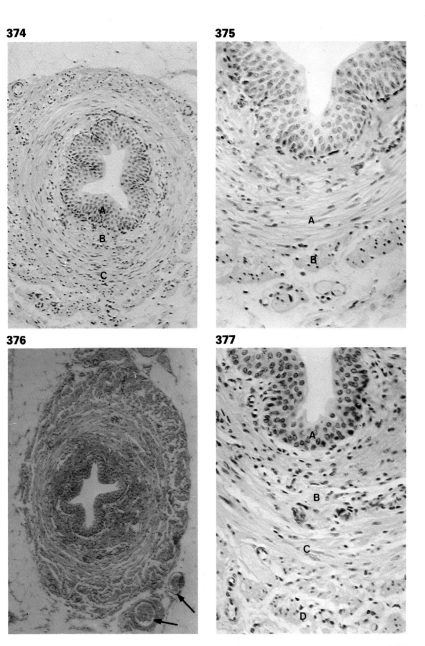

374

375

376

377

223

378 *Urinary bladder (H & E)* The bladder is lined by transitional epithelium (A) resting on a corium (B). A submucosa (C) is also present. The smooth muscle coat (D) is in longitudinal, circular and longitudinal layers. An outer fibrous coat covered by serosa (E) completes the layers.

379 *Urinary bladder (H & E)* High power of **378** to show the corium (A), submucosa (B) and the inner longitudinal muscle coat (C). A group of parasympathetic ganglion cells is present (D).

380 *Urinary bladder (H & E)* High power of **378** to show the mucosa. The lining epithelium (A) is transitional and rests on a corium (B) of loose connective tissue which in turn lies on a submucosa (C) of denser connective tissue.

381 *Urinary bladder (H & E)* High power of **378** to show the outer longitudinal (A) coat of smooth muscle. The fibrous coat (B) is covered by serosal endothelium (C).

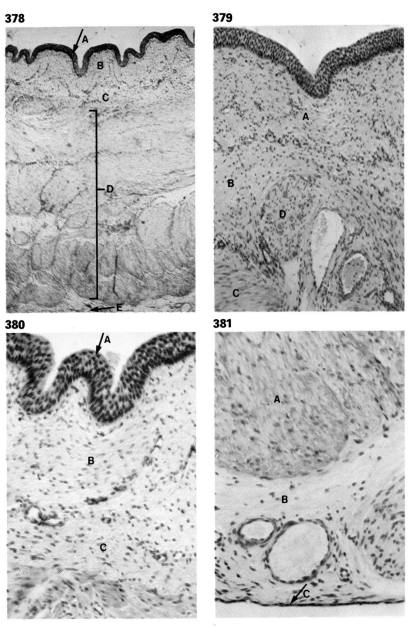

225

382 *Urethra (H & E)* This section passes through the commencement of the urethra in the female. The lumen is collapsed and the smooth muscle of the internal sphincter surrounds it.

383 *Urethra (H & E)* High power of **382** to show transitional epithelium (A) and circular (B) and longitudinal (C) smooth muscle.

382

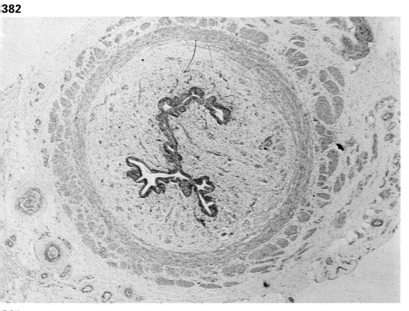

383

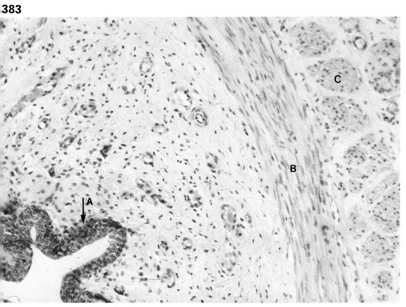

The Male Reproductive System

THE TESTIS

The testis is an endocrine and an exocrine gland of compound tubular type. It lies in the scrotum, which is covered in hairy pigmented skin containing sebaceous glands, smooth muscle (dartos) and skeletal muscle (cremaster). The testis is covered by the endothelium of the visceral layer of the tunica vaginalis testis, deep to which is a thick fibrous capsule (the tunica albuginea). This sends septa into the testicular substance dividing it into lobules. The septa converge on the back of the testis where they form a trabecular network (mediastium testis). Within the lobules lie some 50–100 seminiferous tubules each of which is highly coiled and about a metre in length when unravelled.

The seminiferous tubules are lined by a unique type of stratified epithelium resting on a well-defined basement membrane and containing supporting and spermatogenic cells. The supporting cells (of Sertoli) are tall, slender columnar cells with a spherical pale vesicular nucleus located at the base of the cell, and containing a very large and prominent nucleolus. The cytoplasm of the Sertoli cell reaches the tubule lumen. The sides and apex of the cell are studded by recesses occupied by the spermatogenic cells but this cannot be made out under the light microscope.

The spermatogenic cells

Next to the basement membrane lie the spermatogonia which are of two types, depending on their nuclear configuration. Type A spermatogonia have oval or spherical nuclei with one or two nucleoli attached to the nuclear membrane, and fine chromatin granules. Type B spermatogonia have spherical nuclei with one central nucleolus and chromatin granules of varying size. Type A spermatogonia divide mitotically to give rise to daughter cells which either persist as type A spermatogonia or which differentiate to give rise to type B spermatogonia. Type B spermatogonia divide mitotically to give rise to a pair of primary spermatocytes which remain linked by a cytoplasmic bridge since the process of cell division never reaches completion: this fact can be ascertained only at E.M. level, however.

The primary spermatocytes are large cells with large spherical nuclei. They lie nearer the lumen than the spermatogonia. Coiled chromosomes can often be seen in the nuclei of primary spermatocytes since the spermatocyte-pair divides *meiotically* to give rise to four conjoined secondary spermatocytes. These are smaller than the primary spermatocytes and occupy the middle zone of the germinal epithelium. They are seen infrequently, however, since they divide mitotically after a brief interphase to give rise to eight interconnected spermatids. These are small cells with spherical nuclei and lie next to the lumen of the tubule. They metamorphose into spermatozoa, a process designated spermiogenesis and whilst they are doing so they occupy recesses on the surface of a Sertoli cell.

The mature sperm consists of a head and tail. The head consists of a condensed spermatid nucleus covered anteriorly by the acrosomal cap elaborated by the Golgi apparatus of the spermatid. The tail consists of a neck, a middle piece (5–7µ in length) a principal piece (45µ long) and an end piece (5µ in length). The tail is seen under the electron microscope to have the core of two central hollow fibrils with nine surrounding doublets common to all motile cilia: the peripheral portion of the middle piece contains mitochondria in helical formation and the peripheral part of the principal piece has dense fibres arranged radially.

In man, six clearly-defined stages constitute the cycle of the seminiferous epithelium. Each stage extends over a small sector of the wall so that in any given profile of a seminiferous tubule, whether cut transversely or longitudinally, the appearance of the wall varies from area to area.

In the mediastinum, the seminiferous tubule straightens and joins with its fellows to form a network of anastomosing tubules known as the rete testis and lined by simple squamous epithelium. The rete is drained by the efferent ductules which run into the head of the epididymis and which will be described later under epididymis.

The interstitial tissue

The endocrine portion of the testis is composed of the interstitial tissue lying between the seminiferous tubules. It is composed of loose connective tissue containing blood and lymphatic vessels, nerves and clumps of epithelial cells, the interstitial cells of Leydig. These are the source of the hormone testosterone and have a characteristically vacuolated cytoplasm (cf. adrenal cortex and corpus luteum) in ordinary histological preparations in which fat has been dissolved. Their cytoplasm contains rod-shaped crystalloids (of Reinke). The cells are seen with the E.M. to be rich in agranular endoplasmic reticulum.

THE EPIDIDYMIS

The major portion of the head of the epididymis comprises the efferent ductules. There are about a dozen such tubules connecting the rete testis with the duct of the epididymis. They have a unique epithelial lining which fluctuates between simple low columnar and simple tall columnar. Some of the cells are ciliated. The epithelium rests on loose connective tissue and some circular smooth muscle is present outside this.

The body and tail of the epididymis are composed of the highly coiled *duct of the epididymis* which is about 7m long when unravelled. It is lined by pseudo-stratified ciliated columnar epithelium: there are basal cells and tall columnar epithelial cells with a tuft of non-motile cilia. These last are seen with the E.M. to be very long microvilli, often branched near their bases. The epithelium rests on a corium of loose connective tissue, outside which is some circular smooth muscle. The lumen is packed with spermatozoa.

THE VAS DEFERENS

The wall of this structure is very thick relative to the size of the lumen. It is lined by pseudo-stratified columnar epithelium resting on a delicate basement membrane. The epithelium is ciliated in the extra-abdominal portion of the vas. The corium is of loose connective tissue rich in elastic fibres, and the mucosa is thrown into longitudinal folds, so that the lumen is stellate. It contains a mass of packed spermatozoa. The muscularis is very thick and composed of inner longitudinal, middle circular and outer longitudinal layers of smooth muscle. A fibrous adventitial coat is present. The ampulla of the vas deferens has the same histological appearance as the seminal vesicle.

THE SEMINAL VESICLES

The seminal vesicles, the ampulla of the vas deferens and the ejaculatory ducts have a histological appearance in common. They are lined by pseudo-stratified columnar epithelium resting on a corium of loose connective tissue. The mucosa is characteristically thrown into folds which anastomose so that the lumen is compartmentalised. Circular smooth muscle is present, in addition, in the case of the ampulla of the vas and in the seminal vesicle. Spermatozoa are not found in the seminal vesicles.

THE PROSTATE

The prostate is an aggregate of some 50 compound tubulo-alveolar glands embedded in a fibromuscular stroma of smooth muscle and collagen. The alveoli of the gland are of irregular outline, are lined by simple columnar epithelium and contain a granular secretion. The secretion often condenses to form the prostatic concretions, dense ovoids which may be homogeneous or lamellated in appearance. The prostate has a fibrous capsule containing many parasympathetic ganglion cells and a plexus of veins.

In the prostatic substance lie the prostatic urethra, lined by transitional epithelium and the ejaculatory ducts. For the description of these last, see seminal vesicle.

THE PENIS

The penis is covered in thin hairy skin with sebaceous glands. The dermis is thick and contains smooth muscle, the dartos muscle. The bulk of the penis is composed of three elongated masses of erectile tissue. In the dorsal part of the organ lie the paired corpora cavernosa and in the ventral portion is the median corpus spongiosum which surrounds the cavernous urethra. The corpora cavernosa are invested by a dense collagenous capsule. The capsule of the corpus spongiosum is thin and elastic, on the contrary.

The erectile tissue is composed of wide irregular spaces lined by endothelium and separated by collagenous tissue containing some smooth muscle. The arteries supplying the cavernous spaces are coiled—helicine—in the flaccid penis but become straight during erection. They have a thick media and elongated intimal thickenings known as cushions.

The cavernous urethra is lined by stratified columnar epithelium over most of its extent, but near the anterior urethral orifice the epithelium is stratified squamous of the mucous membrane type. The glans penis is the expanded anterior tip of the corpus spongiosum. It is covered by a fold of skin, the prepuce.

384 *Testis (Iron haematoxylin)* The peripheral parts of the field contain seminiferous tubules cut in various planes. In the centre lies the rete testis sectioned transversely (*arrows*).

385 *Testis (H & E)* Seminiferous tubules lie to left and right. In the centre is the rete testis sectioned longitudinally.

386 *Testis (H & E)* High power of **385** showing portions of two seminiferous tubules. The lining epithelium of one is totally different from that of the other, indicating that the tubules are at different stages of the seminiferous cycle.

387 *Testis (H & E)* High power of **385** to show a single seminiferous tubule in transverse section. Sertoli cell nuclei (A) lie against the basement membrane. The spermatogonia are mostly dividing (B). Primary spermatocyte nuclei (C) and spermatid nuclei (D) are also numerous.

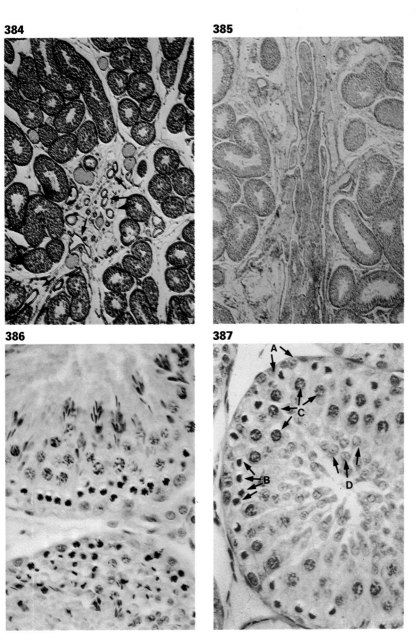

388 *Testis (Iron haematoxylin)* High power of **384** to show portions of four seminiferous tubules with interstitial connective tissue (A) and interstitial cells of Leydig (B) between.

389 *Testis (Iron haematoxylin)* High power of **384** to show portions of two seminiferous tubules in which the epithelium appears similar, indicating that the tubules are in the same stage of the seminiferous cycle.

390 *Testis (Iron haematoxylin)* High power of **384** to show the wall of a seminiferous tubule. Sertoli cells (A) and spermatogonia (B) lie next to the basement membrane. Dividing primary spermatocytes lie at C and spermatids at D.

391 *Testis (Iron haematoxylin)* Part of the wall of a seminiferous tubule and interstitial tissue occupy the field. Four clumps of interstitial cells of Leydig lie in the connective tissue.

388

389

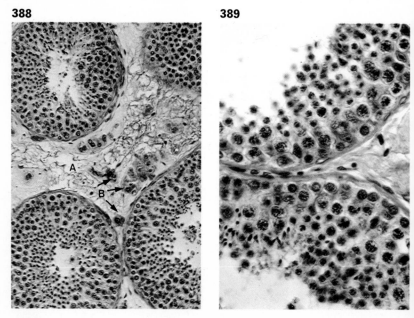

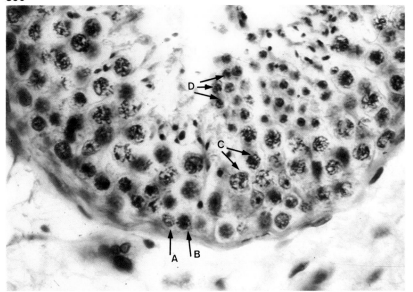

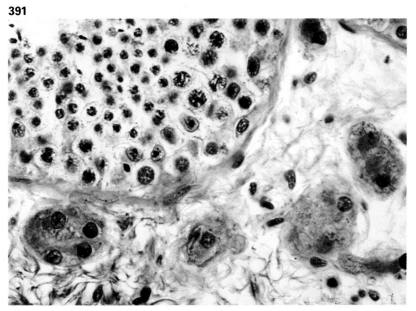

392 *Rete testis (H & E)* In this field the tubules of the rete have been sectioned longitudinally. They are lined by simple squamous epithelium.

393 *Rete testis (H & E)* The tubules of the rete have been sectioned transversely and have simple squamous or cubical epithelium.

394 *Efferent ductule (H & E)* The efferent ductules connect the rete testis with the duct of the epididymis. They are lined by an epithelium which undulates between low and high columnar. Some of the cells are ciliated.

392

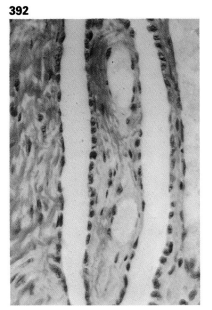

393

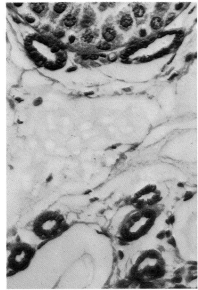

394

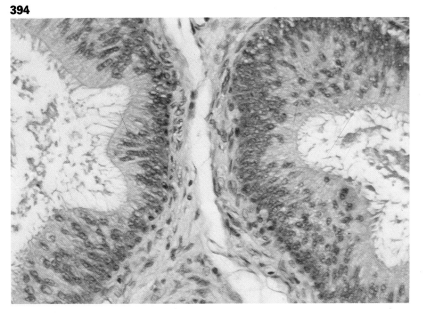

395 *Duct of epididymis (H & E)* The duct of the epididymis is highly coiled and the lumen is packed with spermatozoa.

396 *Duct of epididymis (H & E)* High power of **395** to show the pseudo-stratified ciliated columnar epithelium lining the duct of the epididymis. Some circular smooth muscle is present outside the epithelium (A). The mass of spermatozoa in the lumen can be seen at B.

397 *Duct of epididymis (H & E)* In the tail of the epididymis the duct of the epididymis becomes very thick-walled and lined by pseudo-stratified columnar epithelium—that is it assumes the guise of the vas deferens. In this field the upper three profiles are of the duct as found in the body and the lowest profile of the duct in the tail.

398 *Spermatic cord (Weigert's elastic)* The spermatic cord is a composite of arteries, veins, nerves, skeletal muscle (A) (cremaster), and the vas deferens (B), invested by fascia (C).

399 *Vas deferens (Weigert's elastic)* The corium of the vas (*arrowed*) is rich in elastic fibres.

395

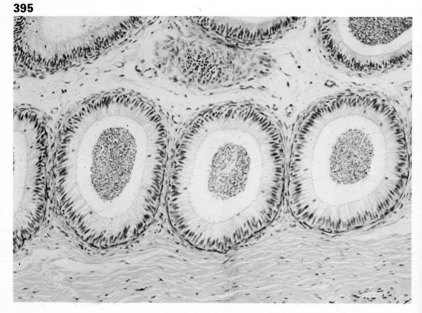

396

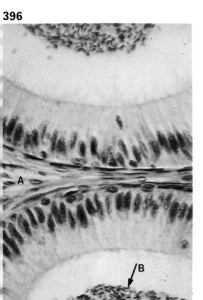

A

B

397

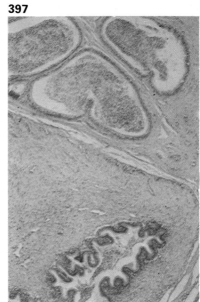

398

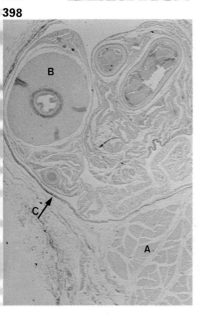

B

C

A

399

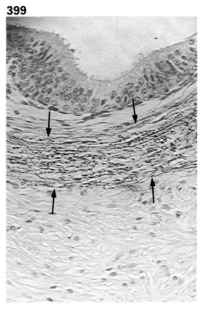

400 *Vas deferens (H & E)* The vas has a stellate lumen and a very thick wall composed largely of smooth muscle.

401 *Vas deferens (H & E)* High power of **400** to show the pseudo-stratified columnar epithelial lining.

402 *Ampulla of vas (H & E)* This portion of the vas has a mucosa which is thrown into folds which anastomose.

403 *Ejaculatory ducts (H & E)* This section through the prostate shows the alveoli of the gland (*bottom*) and the paired ejaculatory ducts (*top*). They have a mucosa which is thrown into anastomosing folds.

404 *Seminal vesicle (H & E)* The mucosa of the seminal vesicle is also thrown into anastomosing folds.

405 *Seminal vesicle (H & E)* High power of **404** to show the mucosal folds. They are covered in simple columnar epithelium and have a core of loose connective tissue. Smooth muscle is present at A.

400

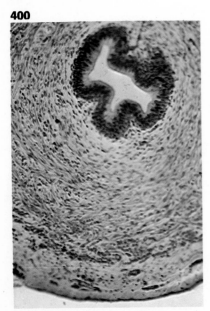

401

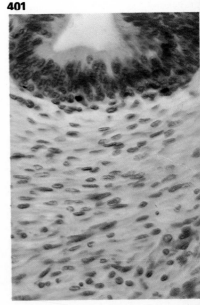

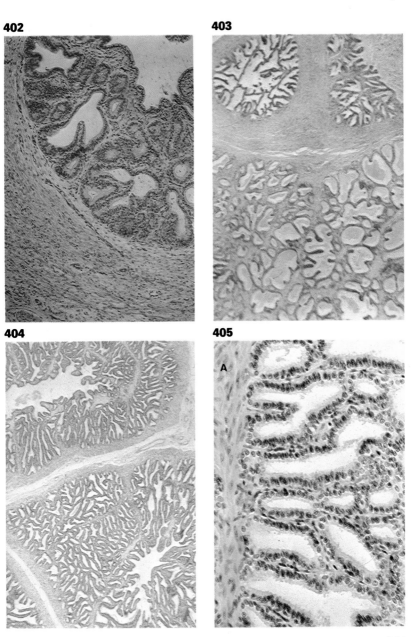

406 *Prostate (H & E)* The gland is composed of irregular alveoli embedded in a fibromuscular stroma, but with this stain both the collagen and smooth muscle of the stroma stain pink. Two concretions are in the field (*arrows*).

407 *Prostate (Masson)* Smooth muscle is stained purple and collagen is stained green by this method. The fibromuscular stroma is therefore well demonstrated. A single concretion is present in one alveolus (*arrow*).

408 *Prostate (H & E)* High power of **406** to show prostatic alveoli lined by simple columnar epithelium.

409 *Prostate (H & E)* A concretion is present in both alveoli in this field from a human prostate. The lower concretion is homogeneous but the upper is slightly lamellated.

410 *Prostate (H & E)* The urethra (prostatic portion), passes through the substance of the prostate and lies in the upper right corner of this field.

411 *Prostate (H & E)* High power of **410** to show the urethral wall. The lining epithelium is transitional.

406

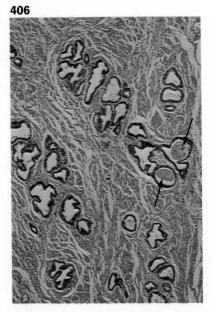

407

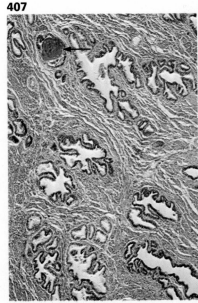

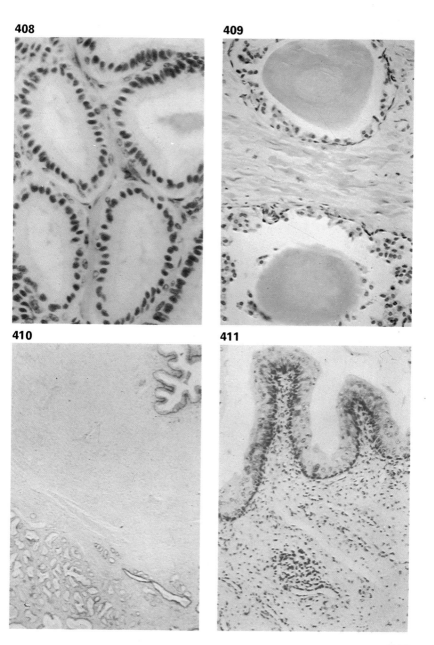

408

409

410

411

243

412 *Prostate (H & E)* The capsule of the gland. It is collagenous and contains many groups of parasympathetic ganglion cells (*arrows*).

413 *Prostate (H & E)* High power of **412** to show a group of parasympathetic ganglion cells.

414 *TS penis (H & E)* The penis is covered by epidermis (A). On the dorsum are the paired corpora cavernosa (B) and ventrally lies the corpus spongiosum (C) with the cavernous urethra (D) in its substance.

415 *Penis (H & E)* High power of the corpus spongiosum from **414**. It is composed of cavernous tissue with the urethra running through. The urethra is lined by stratified columnar epithelium.

416 *Penis (H & E)* High power of a corpus cavernosum from **414**. It is invested by a tough collagenous capsule (A) and is composed of erectile tissue.

417 *Penis (H & E)* High power of the cavernous erectile tissue of the corpus cavernosum. The tissue is composed of vascular spaces lined by endothelium with connective tissue and smooth muscle between.

412

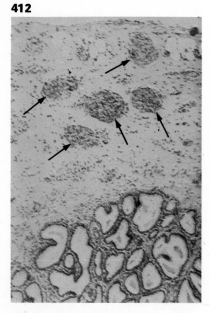

413

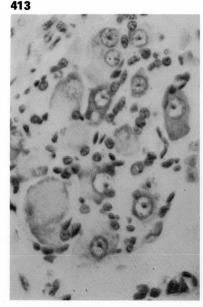

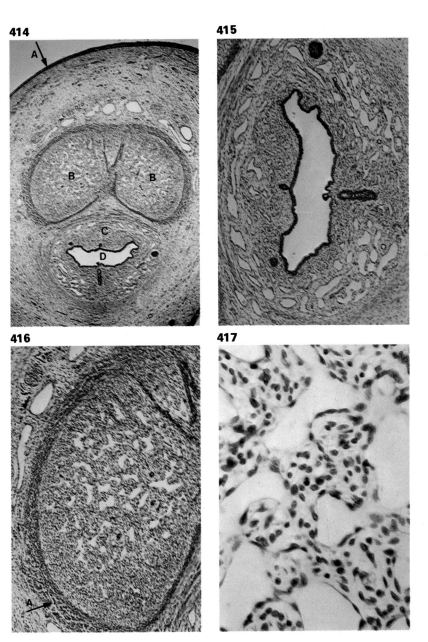

245

The Female Reproductive System

THE OVARY

The ovary, like the testis, is at one and the same time an endocrine and an exocrine gland: the hormones it produces are oestrogens and progesterone.

The ovary is divided into a medulla and a cortex. The medulla is composed of areolar connective tissue containing many blood vessels, nerves and lymphatic vessels. The ovary is covered by a simple cubical (germinal) epithelium, deep to which is a tunica albuginea of dense fibrous tissue.

The ovarian cortex is composed of a highly cellular stroma of loose connective tissue and contains the ovarian follicles. The ovarian follicles may be resting (primordial), maturing or mature (Graafian).

The primordial follicles
These lie just deep to the tunica albuginea and are composed of a single primary oocyte of 25μ diameter, surrounded by a single layer of squamous epithelial cells—the follicular epithelium.

The maturing follicles
In these the ovum, the follicular epithelium and the ovarian stroma all become involved in the maturation process. The ovum, or primary oocyte increases in diameter to more than 100 microns. It comes to be surrounded by a homogeneous membrane, the zona pellucida. The follicular epithelium undergoes mitosis and becomes multilayered, the cells altering shape concomitantly from squamous to polyhedral. The ovarian stroma condenses to form the theca folliculi, which is arranged in inner cellular and outer fibrous layers. The cells of the inner layer of the theca acquire a yellow pigment in their cytoplasm and are known as theca lutein cells. They produce the hormone progesterone.

The Graafian follicles
A fluid-filled cavity, the antrum, appears amongst the follicular epithelial cells and gradually expands until the ovum is pushed to the side wall of an enormous cyst lined by the follicular epithelial cells. The lining epithelium is designated the membrana granulosa as the epithelial cells now have a granular cytoplasm. The ovum, with a covering of follicular epithelium, projects (cumulus oophorus) into the antrum. A fully mature follicle occupies the whole thickness of the cortex eventually.

The mature Graafian follicle finally comes to bulge the ovarian surface and ruptures. The ovum, surrounded by a few layers of follicular epithelial cells (corona radiata) is discharged into the peritoneal cavity. The wall of the follicle becomes folded, and the follicle becomes converted to an endocrine gland, the corpus luteum. Twelve hours before ovulation the primary oocyte completes the meiotic division into a secondary oocyte and a first polar body.

The corpus luteum
The epithelial cells of the membrana granulosa become enlarged (up to 25

microns across) and are known as granulosa lutein cells. The basement membrane between the membrana granulosa and the theca disappears and capillaries grow in from the theca. The granulosa lutein cells produce both oestrogen and progesterone and so acquire a foamy cytoplasm in ordinary H & E preparations. Like the theca lutein cells, they have a yellow pigment in their cytoplasm. The corpus luteum degenerates in 10–14 days if fertilisation does not occur. If pregnancy supervenes the corpus luteum persists for several months and attains a size of some 2–3cm. The corpus luteum in either case eventually degenerates and is replaced by a scar, the corpus albicans.

THE UTERINE TUBE

This tubular structure connects the peritoneal cavity with the uterine lumen. The lateral extremity, or infundibulum is drawn out into many finger-like projections, the fimbriae. The main portion of the uterine tube is the ampulla. As it approaches the uterus the uterine tube narrows, to form the isthmus. Finally the uterine tube negotiates the wall of the body of the uterus—the intramural portion. The isthmus and intramural portion have a similar structure which differs from that of the ampulla.

The ampulla of the uterine tube
The lining epithelium is simple columnar. The cells lie in alternating groups of ciliated and non-ciliated type. Outside the epithelium is a corium of highly cellular loose connective tissue. The mucosa is thrown into folds which in the ampulla branch extensively but which in the isthmus are less branched: the lumen is almost completely obliterated in the process. Outside the mucosa is a muscularis of spiral smooth muscle. A serosa is present on the outside.

The intramural portion of the uterine tube
This part of the tube bears a close resemblance to the vas deferens. The lumen is stellate. The lining is of non-ciliated and ciliated columnar epithelial cell clumps alternating with one another. The corium is again of very cellular loose connective tissue. The muscularis is very thick, being the myometrium of the uterus.

THE UTERUS

The wall of the uterus is composed of a mucous membrane (endometrium) resting directly on a very thick smooth muscle coat (myometrium) with a fibrous adventitia outside this. A serous coat will be present additionally in the case of the body of the uterus. The mucous membrane of the cervix of the uterus does not undergo changes in morphology during the menstrual cycle, unlike the mucosa of the body.

The body of the uterus

The endometrium of the body can be subdivided into a superficial pars functionalis which is shed during menstruation and a deep pars basalis which is not. The lining epithelium of the uterus is simple columnar. Simple test-tube glands also lined by simple columnar epithelium occur in the endometrium. The corium is of highly cellular loose connective tissue. After menstruation the epithelial cells lining the stumps of the glands in the pars basalis proliferate in order to re-epithelialise the raw endometrial surface. This proliferative phase lasts until mid-cycle and during this time the endometrium attains a height of some 2mm.

After mid-cycle the endometrium enters the progestational (secretory) phase, during which the endometrium increases in height from 2 to about 5mm. The glands become highly coiled and saw-toothed in appearance. Their lining cells acquire large deposits of lipid and glycogen in their cytoplasm. Arterioles can be seen spiralling between the glands towards the surface. The deeper part of the pars functionalis becomes highly oedematous and dilated lymphatic vessels are found: this part of the functionalis is now designated the stratum spongiosum. The superficial part of the functionalis remains compact as the stratum compactum.

During the menstrual phase the pars functionalis is shed, accompanied by haemorrhage, but no clotting occurs. The pars basalis, containing the stumps of the glands, alone remains, and the cycle re-commences.

The myometrium is composed of smooth muscle bundles running in all directions with loose connective tissue, and large blood vessels and nerves between. A serous coat of endothelial cells resting on loose connective tissue is present on the outside except along the line of attachment of the broad ligament.

The cervix of the uterus

The cervix differs from the body in several respects. The lining epithelium is mucus-secreting, and the glands are larger and branched. Their lining cells also secrete mucus. The endometrial stroma is less cellular than that of the body, and the myometrium is not so thick. A serosa is present only on the upper cervix. At the external os there is an abrupt change from simple columnar to the stratified squamous epithelium of the vagina.

THE EXTERNAL GENITALIA

The vagina

The vagina is lined by a mucous membrane composed of stratified squamous epithelium resting on a highly vascular corium of loose connective tissue. Outside this is some smooth muscle arranged for the most part in a longitudinal direction although some circular fibres do occur. A fibrous adventitial coat is present.

The greater vestibular glands (of Bartholin)
These are compound tubulo-alveolar mucus-secreting glands. The ducts of the gland are lined by simple cubical epithelium.

The labia minora
These are mucosal folds. They are covered by stratified squamous epithelium of the mucous membrane variety, and have a corium of loose connective tissue. Sebaceous glands opening directly to the surface are found.

The labia majora
These are folds of skin. They are covered by pigmented epidermis and possess hair follicles, sebaceous and sweat glands on their outer aspect only.

The clitoris
This is covered in stratified squamous epithelium of mucous membrane type. In the loose connective tissue core of the organ lie masses of erectile tissue analagous with the corpora cavernosa of the penis. Many large nerve bundles are present in the corium.

THE PLACENTA

The placenta is smooth and shiny on its foetal aspect where it is covered by a layer of simple cubical epithelium, the amniotic epithelium. This rests on a layer of embryonic connective tissue (or mesenchyme) known as the chorion. The bulk of the placenta is composed of chorionic villi of foetal origin and lying in a lake of maternal blood. The villi are covered by trophoblast and have a core of mesenchyme containing foetal blood vessels. The covering trophoblast is arranged in superficial syncytial and deep cellular layers. The appearance of the chorionic villi alters as the placenta develops.

Chorionic villi in the early placenta
These are covered externally by a thick layer of syncytiotrophoblast, a multinucleate mass of basophilic cytoplasm. Deep to this the trophoblast is arranged as one or two layers of cubical cells. The foetal blood vessels lie near the centre of the villus and contain erythrocytes which are usually nucleated.

Chorionic villi in late placentae
The syncytiotrophoblast is now arranged in thick (14–16μ) regions (syncytial knots) alternating with thin (2–14μ) areas: these latter are seen with the E.M. to be richly endowed with microvilli and are believed to be involved in placental transport. The thick portions are believed to be concerned with synthesis and secretion of the placental hormones (oestrogen, progesterone, lactogen and chorionic gonadotrophin). Deep to the syncytium is the cytotrophoblast, but now found as an occasional cell here and there. The foetal blood vessels lie in

the periphery of the villi, adjacent to the regions of thin syncytiotrophoblast. Their contained erythrocytes are usually anucleate.

The maternal component of the placenta comprises the endometrium deep to the implantation site, now known as the decidua basalis. The stromal connective tissue cells have hypertrophied to become large and irregular and have proliferated so as to be very numerous. They are known as decidual cells, may be binucleate, and may contain large amounts of glycogen.

THE UMBILICAL CORD

The umbilical cord is covered in the simple cubical epithelium of the amnion. Its core is composed of mesenchyme (Wharton's jelly) embedded in which are the paired umbilical arteries and one umbilical vein. The umbilical arteries lack an internal elastic lamina and a tunica adventitia. Their tunica media is arranged in inner longitudinal and outer circular layers of smooth muscle.

THE MAMMARY GLAND

The breast is a compound of some 15–20 modified sweat glands embedded in an interlobular stroma of dense fibro-fatty tissue. Each lobule of the gland is formed by a compound tubulo-alveolar gland opening at the nipple by means of a long lactiferous duct lined by stratified cubical epithelium. The intralobular connective tissue is loose and cellular, however. Myoepithelial cells are present.

The gland parenchyma shows wide variations according to the age and

continued

418 *Ovary (H & E)* This ovary, from a small mammal, exhibits cortex (A) and medulla (B). The cortex contains ovarian follicles in varying stages of development. A corpus luteum is also present (C).

419 *Ovary (H & E)* Medium power view of ovarian cortex showing primordial follicles (A) and early (B) maturing follicles.

420 *Ovary (H & E)* The germinal epithelium (A) covering the ovary is simple cubical. Deep to it is the tunica albuginea (B). A primordial follicle (C) has a central ovum surrounded by a single layer of flattened follicular epithelium.

421 *Ovary (Azan)* The tunica albuginea is well illustrated by this staining method in which collagen fibres are stained bright blue. The germinal epithelium is at A and a primordial follicle lies at B.

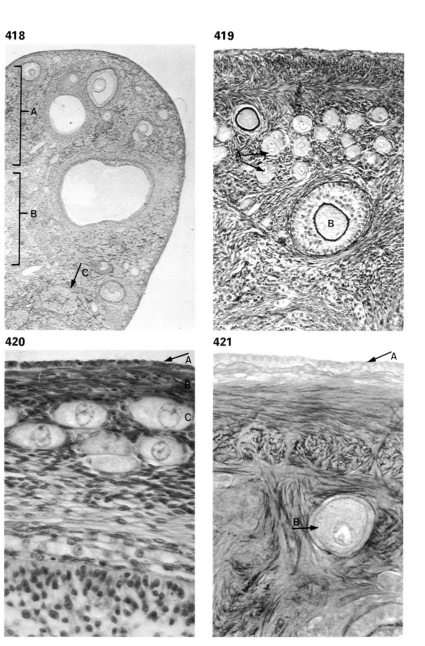

418

419

420

421

condition of the person. Three distinct states occur, prelactating, lactating, and post-lactating.

The pre-lactation gland

The mammary gland is rudimentary prior to its first lactation. It is a compound tubular gland until then. The terminal tubules of the gland are lined by a simple cubical epithelium.

The lactating gland

During pregnancy the mammary gland completes its differentiation. The terminal tubules form buds which expand into alveoli. At the end of the pregnancy the alveoli are large and of irregular outline and lined by cubical or low columnar epithelium. The lobules vary widely in activity. The cells in an actively secreting lobule will contain large apical fat droplets in many instances and the lumen of the lobule will contain a secretion of very heterogenous nature being composed of droplets of fat, cytoplasmic debris and desquamated cells. The ducts of the gland will contain a similar secretion.

The post-lactation gland

After pregnancy the gland slowly reverts to the compound tubular state, the alveoli decreasing in size until they are no longer distinguishable.

The nipple is surrounded by the areola, a region of pigmented epidermis. The dermis of the areola contains circular smooth muscle which on contraction causes erection. Many sebaceous glands lie in the nipple. Around the periphery of the areola are sweat glands (of Montgomery) which cause surface elevations. The nipple contains the lactiferous sinus, a dilatation which receives the ducts of the individual lobules of the gland.

---

422 *Ovary (H & E)* A ripening follicle from **418**. The nucleus (A) and cytoplasm (B) of the ovum are surrounded by the zona pellucida (C) and a row of polyhedral follicular epithelial cells (D). The stroma is beginning to condense around the follicle as the theca (E).

423 *Ovary (Azan)* An early Graafian follicle is shown. The follicular epithelium is now stratified (A) and liquor is starting to appear (B). The stromal condensation to form the theca is now well advanced (C).

424 *Ovary (Azan)* High power of **423** to show the ovum (A), zona pellucida (B), follicular epithelium (C), and theca (D).

425 *Ovary (H & E)* A Graafian follicle of an intermediate stage of development. The antrum is now of some size and the ovum is displaced to one side.

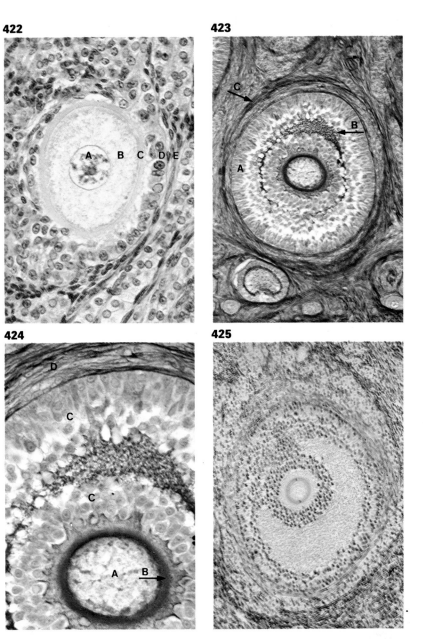

426 *Ovary (Azan)* A Graafian follicle at an intermediate stage of development is again shown. The liquor folliculi stains bright blue with Azan.

427 *Ovary (Azan)* High power of **426** to show the nucleus (A), and cytoplasm, now highly vacuolated (B), of the ovum. The zona pellucida (C), follicular epithelium (D), and liquor folliculi (E) are also illustrated.

428 *Ovary (H & E)* A fully-developed Graafian follicle forms, as here, a conspicuous bulge on the ovarian surface (*arrows*).

429 *Ovary (H & E)* High power of **428** to show the ovum (A) surrounded by the zona pellucida (B) and the columnar follicular epithelial cells known as the corona radiata (C).

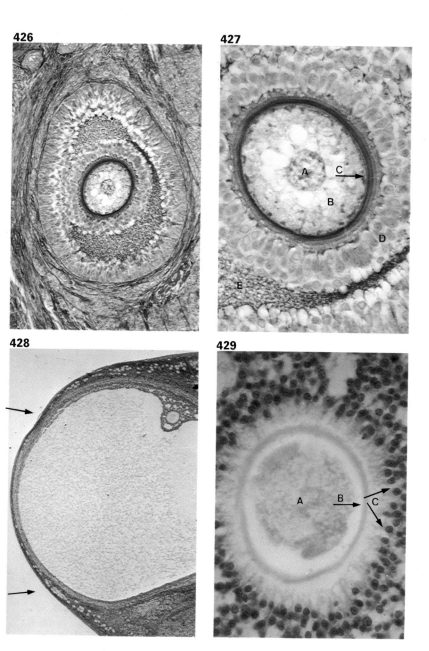

255

430 *Ovary (H & E)* An early corpus luteum from **418**. The structure is highly folded since it is derived from the collapse of a Graafian follicle. The cells of the corpus are of thecal origin and are known as theca lutein cells.

431 *Ovary (H & E)* Low power view of an ovary from a small mammal showing a fully-developed corpus luteum (*arrows*).

432 *Ovary (H & E)* High power view of part of a corpus luteum of pregnancy. The epithelial cells are large and characteristically have a vacuolated cytoplasm in standard histological preparations since the steroid hormones have dissolved.

433 *Ovary (Azan)* High power view of a portion of a corpus luteum of pregnancy to show the granulosa lutein cells. They are large and their cytoplasm is vacuolated.

434 *Ovary and fimbria of uterine tube (H & E)* The fimbriated portion of the uterine tube is seen (*top*) overhanging the ovary.

435 *Ampulla of uterine tube (H & E)* The mucosa of the uterine tube is thrown into folds which are of such complexity as to reduce the lumen to a mere slit. Circular smooth muscle surrounds the mucosa at A.

430

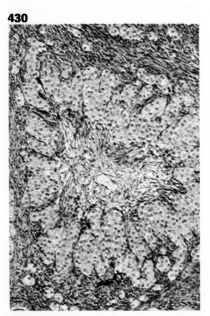

431

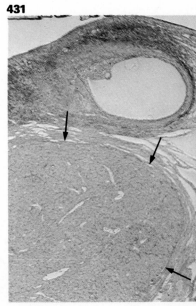

432

433

434

435

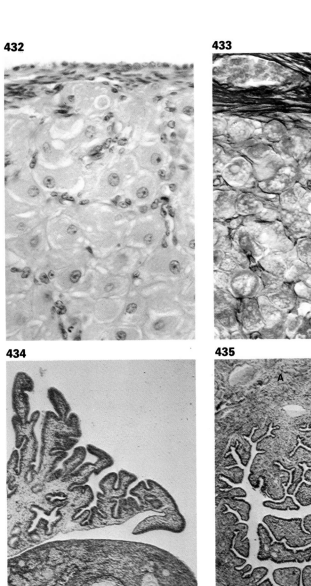

436 *Ampulla of uterine tube (H & E)* High power of **435** to show the simple columnar epithelial lining of the uterine tube. Some of the cells are ciliated.

437 *Isthmus of uterine tube (H & E)* The part of the uterine tube near the wall of the uterus is shown here. The mucosal folds are much less elaborate and the lumen is now wide and of stellate outline.

438 *Body of uterus, menstrual phase (H & E)* The endometrium occupies most of the field but a small portion of the myometrium lies at the foot of the picture. The superficial part of the endometrium has started to break down.

439 *Body of uterus, proliferative phase (H & E)* The endometrium lies in the upper half of the picture and the myometrium in the lower.

440 *Body of uterus, proliferative phase (H & E)* High power of the endometrium from **439**. The lining epithelium is simple columnar and dips in to form short test-tube glands. The stroma is highly cellular.

441 *Body of uterus (H & E)* High power of the myometrium from **439**. It is composed of smooth muscle fibres running in all directions.

436

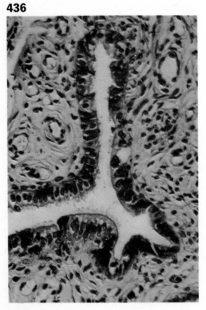

437

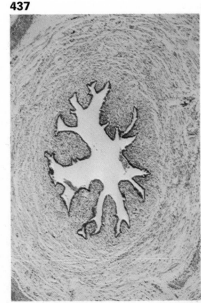

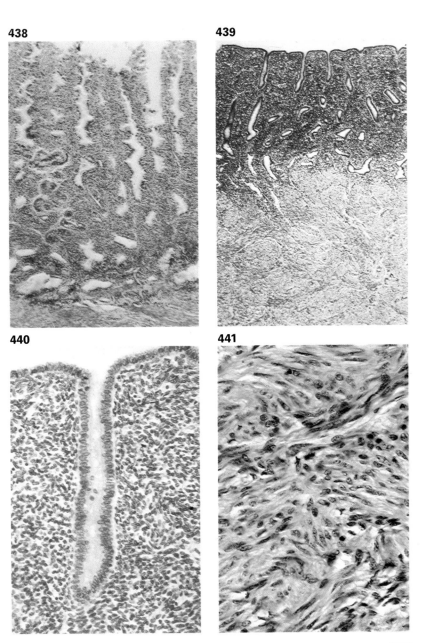

438

439

440

441

259

442 *Body of uterus, progestational phase (H & E)* The endometrium is now subdivisible into an outer stratum compactum (A), a middle stratum spongiosum (B), and a deep pars basalis (C). The myometrium is at D.

443 *Body of uterus, progestational phase (H & E)* Higher power view of figure **442** to show saw-tooth glands (A), a spiral arteriole (B), and a cyst (C).

444 *Body of uterus, progestational phase (H & E)* High power of **442** showing a spiral arteriole (A) and dilated lymphatic vessels filled with exudate (B).

445 *Body of uterus, progestational phase (H & E)* High power of **442** to show a uterine gland with typical saw-tooth outline.

446 *TS cervix of uterus (H & E)* The glands of the cervix are compound— i.e. they branch, as opposed to the glands of the body which do not.

447 *TS cervix of uterus (Mucicarmine)* The same cervix as in **446** is here stained to show the mucous content of the lining epithelial cells.

442

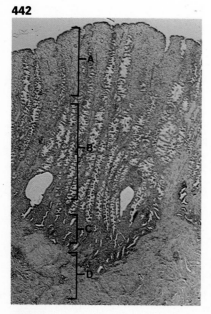

443

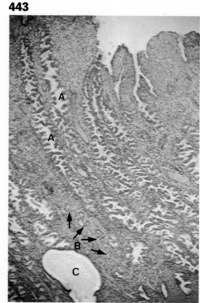

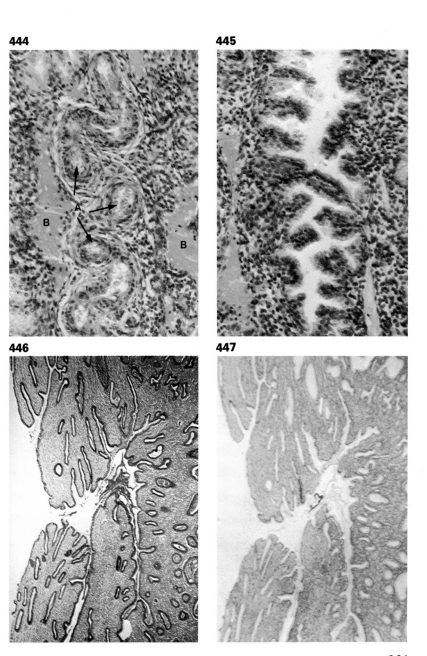

448 *Cervix of uterus (H & E)* High power view of a field from **446** to show a branching cervical gland lined by simple columnar epithelium.

449 *Cervix of uterus (Mucicarmine)* High power of **447** to show a branching cervical gland whose lining epithelium is rich in mucus.

450 *Vagina (H & E)* The vagina is lined by a mucosa consisting of stratified squamous epithelium (A), resting on a corium (B) of loose connective tissue. Outside this is a muscularis (C) of smooth muscle and a fibrous adventitia (D).

451 *Vagina (H & E)* High power of **450** to show the stratified squamous epithelium of the vagina.

452 *Glands of Bartholin (H & E)* These glands are of compound tubulo-alveolar type and are mucus-secreting.

453 *Glands of Bartholin (H & E)* High power of **452** to show three alveoli lined by a simple mucus-secreting columnar epithelium and a duct lined by simple cubical epithelium.

448

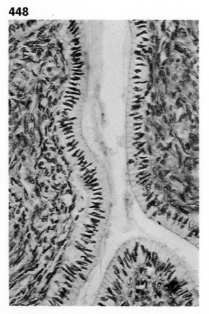

449

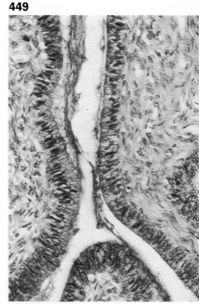

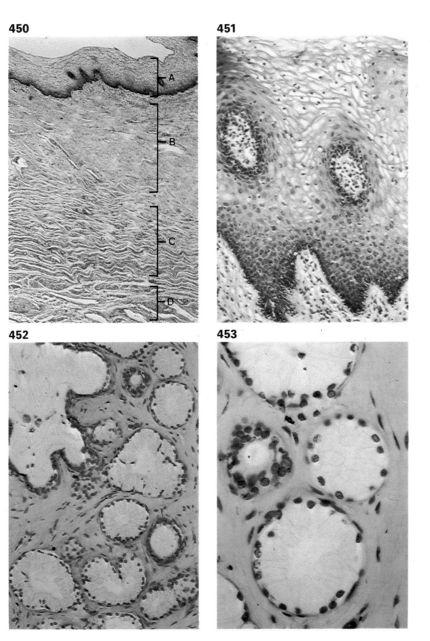

450

451

452

453

263

454 *Clitoris and labia minora (H & E)* The clitoris (A) is flanked by the labia minora (B). A part of a labium majus is seen (C).

455 *Clitoris (H & E)* The clitoris is covered by stratified squamous epithelium and contains cavernous erectile tissue and large nerves.

456 *Clitoris (H & E)* High power of **455** to show stratified squamous epithelium (A), erectile tissue (B), and large nerves (C).

457 *Clitoris (H & E)* The endothelial-lined vascular spaces of the erectile tissue are seen at A and several large nerves are also seen (B).

458 *Labium minus (H & E)* High power of **454** to show a labium minus. It is covered in stratified squamous epithelium of the mucous membrane variety and has sebaceous glands opening directly to the surface.

459 *Labium minus (H & E)* High power of **458** to show the stratified squamous epithelium and sebaceous glands.

454

455

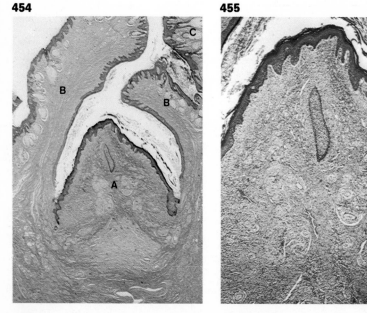

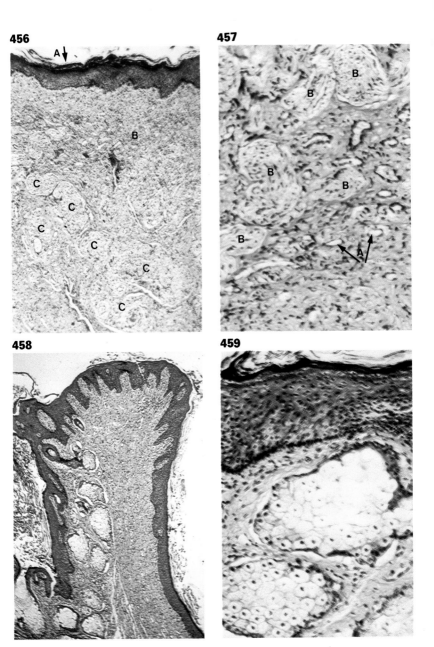

460 *Labium majus (H & E)* The labia majora are folds of skin, and have hair follicles with their associated sebaceous glands.

461 *Labium majus (H & E)* High power of **460** to show the epidermis (A), a hair follicle (B) and sebaceous glands (C).

462 *Umbilical cord (H & E)* The cord is covered in amniotic epithelium (A) and contains two umbilical arteries (B) and an umbilical vein (C) embedded in embryonic connective tissue (Wharton's jelly) (D).

463 *Umbilical cord (H & E)* High power of the simple cubical epithelium of the amnion, with embryonic connective tissue underlying it.

464 *Early placenta (H & E)* This human placenta of two months has chorionic villi (A) bathed by a lake of maternal blood (B).

465 *Early placenta (H & E)* High power of a villus from **464**. The covering trophoblast is thick and has outer syncytial (A) and inner cellular (B) layers. The foetal capillaries lie in the centre of the villus.

460

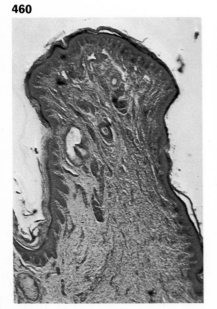

461

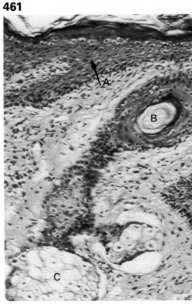

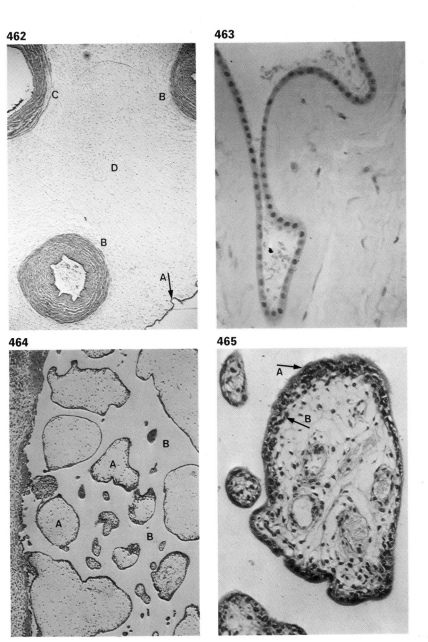

267

466 *Mature placenta (H & OGE)* The field shows a placental septum (*right*) and chorionic villi bathed by maternal blood (*left*).

467 *Mature placenta (H & OGE)* High power of **466** to show a villus. The trophoblastic covering is now thin and composed mainly of syncytium (A) with some cytotrophoblast in places (B). A syncytial knot lies at C. The foetal vessels (D) lie in the periphery of the villus.

468 *Decidua (H & OGE)* The endometrium of the pregnant uterus is known as the decidua. The stromal cells are greatly enlarged and rich in cytoplasmic glycogen.

469 *Inactive mammary gland (H & OGE)* This specimen is from a female who has never been pregnant. The connective tissue stroma (A) of the gland is extensive and the lobules (B) poorly developed. A duct lies at C.

470 *Inactive mammary gland (H & OGE)* High power of **469** to show a lobule of the gland. The alveoli are lined by simple cubical epithelium and can, as here, contain secretion.

466

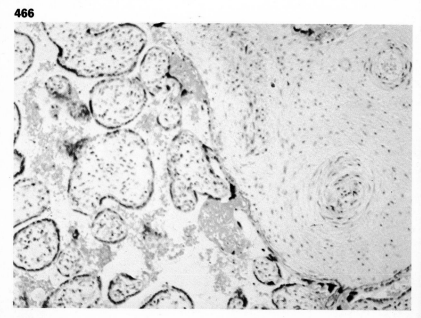

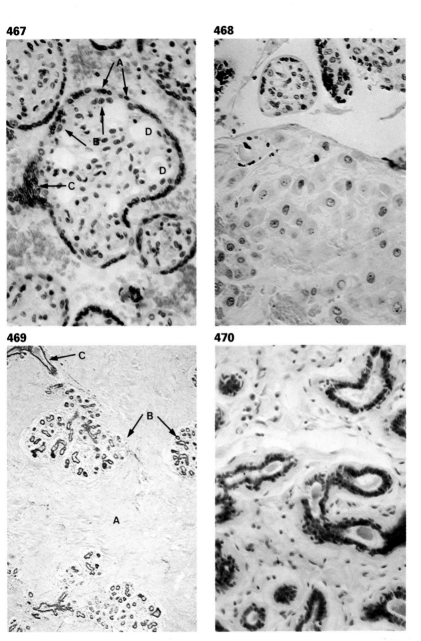

471 *Active mammary gland (H & E)* The lobules of the gland (A) are now extensive and the connective tissue stroma (B) is reduced in amount. Fat cells lie at C and lactiferous ducts at D.

472 *Active mammary gland (H & E)* Medium power view of a lobule from figure **471**. The alveoli (A) and lactiferous ducts (B) have a heterogenous secretion in their lumen.

473 *Active mammary gland (H & E)* High power of **471** to show glandular alveoli (A) filled with heterogenous secretion rich in fatty droplets. The lactiferous duct is lined by stratified cubical epithelium (B).

471

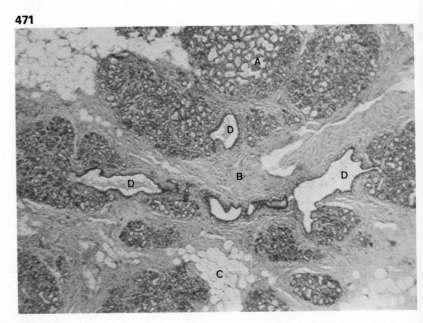

472

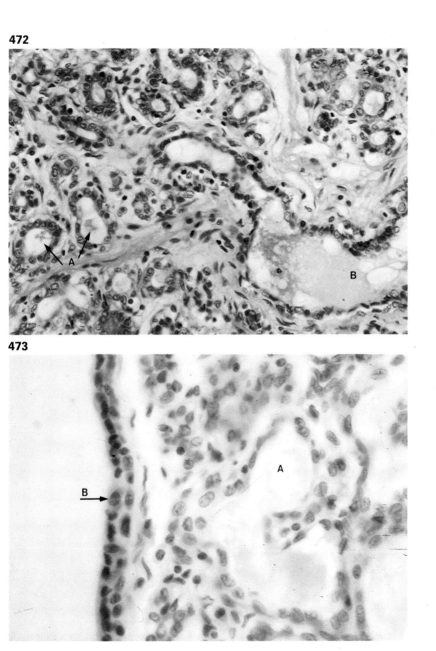

473

271

The Auditory Apparatus

THE EXTERNAL AND MIDDLE EAR

The pinna
The pinna is composed of thin skin containing some hairs, sweat glands and sebaceous glands resting on cartilage of the elastic variety.

The external auditory meatus
This has a wall of elastic cartilage in its outer one-third and of compact bone in its inner two-thirds. It is lined by hairy skin containing sebaceous and ceruminous glands. The ceruminous glands are modified sweat glands of the 'apocrine' type: they are composed of wide tubules lined by a simple squamous or cuboidal epithelium and secrete the wax found in the meatus. They open to the surface by short ducts lined by stratified cubical epithelium.

The tympanic membrane
This is trilaminar. It is covered externally by thin epidermis and internally by the simple cubical epithelium of the middle ear cavity. It has a connective tissue core, the collagenous fibres of which are arranged in outer radial and inner circular layers.

The middle ear cavity or tympanum
This is lined by a simple squamous or simple cubical epithelium resting on a thin lamina propria which blends with the periosteum of the temporal bone. The auditory ossicles, malleus, incus and stapes are composed of compact bone and lack a marrow cavity. The handle of the malleus is attached to the tympanic membrane. The base plate of the stapes has a circumferential fibrous joint connecting it to the margin of the fenestra ovalis (oval window). Two synovial joints join the three ossicles. The tensor tympani and stapedius muscles are skeletal and are attached by tendons to the handle of the malleus and the neck of the stapes respectively. The round window is closed by an elastic (secondary tympanic) membrane. The base plate of the stapes separates the air-filled tympanic cavity from the perilymph in the scala vestibuli of the cochlea. The secondary tympanic membrane separates the tympanum from the perilymph of the scala tympani of the cochlea.

The eustachian (pharyngo-tympanic) tube
This connects the tympanum with the nasopharynx. Its wall is composed of compact bone at its tympanic end and of hyaline cartilage at its pharyngeal extremity. The walls of the latter part are usually in apposition and are separated during the act of swallowing. The tube is lined by simple ciliated columnar epithelium at the middle ear extremity and by pseudo-stratified columnar epithelium with goblet cells at its pharyngeal end. The epithelium rests on a lamina propria of loose connective tissue. The tube serves to equalise the air pressure, at that of the atmosphere, on either side of the ear drum.

THE INNER EAR

The inner ear is composed of the osseous labyrinth and the membranous labyrinth. The two correspond in large measure but differ in points of detail.

The osseous labyrinth
The osseous labyrinth is composed of series of spaces in the petrous portion of the temporal bone. These are: the vestibule, the three bony semicircular canals, and the bony cochlea (i.e. scala vestibuli and scala tympani). The bony labyrinth is lined by endothelium and contains a clear fluid, the perilymph.

The membranous labyrinth
This is suspended from the wall of the bony labyrinth by connective tissue strands over most of its extent but in some places it lies against one side wall of the bony labyrinth. It consists of: the utricle, the utriculo-saccular duct, the saccule, the endolymphatic duct and sac, the three membranous semicircular canals, and the scala media of the cochlea (cochlear duct).

The membranous labyrinth is composed of a connective tissue wall lined by epithelium and contains a clear fluid, the endolymph. The lining epithelium is for the most part simple squamous but may be cubical or columnar in places. In six places, the epithelium is supplanted by neuroepithelial receptor centres of highly unique form and specialised function. They are: a crista in each semicircular canal, a macula in each of the utricle and the saccule, and the organ of Corti in the scala media of the cochlea.

The cristae
One extremity of each semicircular canal has a dilatation (ampulla) housing a crista. This is an elongated ridge projecting into the ampulla at right angles to the long axis of the canal. It is composed of a tall columnar epithelium consisting of two kinds of cells, hair cells and sustentacular cells. The hair cells are flask-shaped and have a basal nucleus. The hairs on their free surface are embedded in a gelatinous mass, the cupula. With the E.M. the hair cells are seen to be of two types and the 'hairs' consist of a single cilium and many modified microvilli. The vestibular nerve sends terminals around the bases of the hair cells. The sustentacular cells are of hour-glass shape with basal nuclei.

The maculae
These bear a close resemblance histologically to the cristae but differ in the respect that they do not project to any great extent into the utricle or saccule, as the case may be. Hair cells and sustentacular cells are again found. The microvilli of the hair cells are embedded in the otolithic membrane: this contains many small crystals of a calcium carbonate-protein complex, which are known as otoliths. The supporting cells are again tall columns.

The three cristae and the two maculae are concerned with the sense of equilibrium, and are associated with the vestibular nerve.

The organ of Corti

This is located in the floor of the cochlear duct and rests on the basilar membrane: it extends from the osseous spiral lamina to the spiral ligament. It is composed of hair cells and supporting cells.

The pillars of Corti are arranged as two rows of cells (the inner and outer pillars) whose nucleated basal portions are wide apart where they rest on the basilar membrane and whose apices are in contact. The pillars thus enclose a triangular space, the inner tunnel, which contains a gelatinous substance and which is crossed by fine transversely-running nerve fibres. Flanking the pillars of Corti lie the hair cells, arranged in a single inner row and in from three to five outer rows. The hair cells are separated from the basilar membrane by supporting cells (of Deiters). The hairs (microvilli) are embedded in the tectorial membrane, a gelatinous mass attached to the osseous spiral lamina. Lateral to the outer hair cells are seven or eight rows of columnar supporting cells. Medial to the inner hair cells are slender border cells which delineate the inner edge of the organ.

---

474 *External auditory meatus (H & E)* The meatus is lined by epidermis (A) and hair follicles (B) and sebaceous glands are present. The ceruminous glands lie at C. This section is through the cartilaginous (outer) part of the meatus, the cartilage (D) being of the elastic type.

475 *External auditory meatus (H & E)* High power of **474** to show the sebaceous glands of the external auditory meatus.

476 *External auditory meatus (H & E)* High power of **474** to show the ceruminous glands (A). They are lined by simple squamous or cubical epithelium and contain wax (B). A duct (C) lined by stratified cubical epithelium is also present.

477 *External auditory meatus (H & E)* High power of **474** to show the elastic cartilage. The elastic fibres in the matrix are not demonstrated by H & E staining.

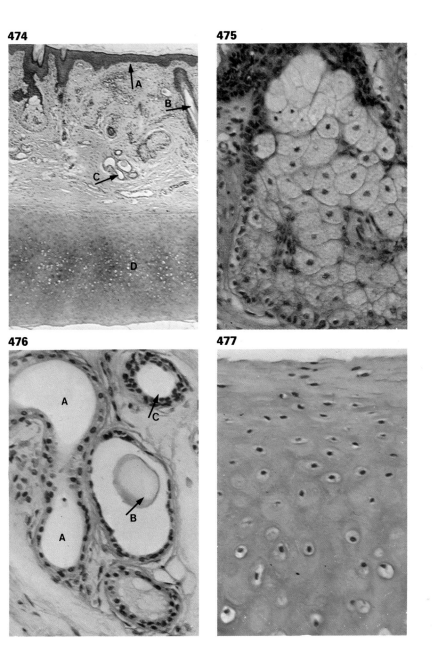

478

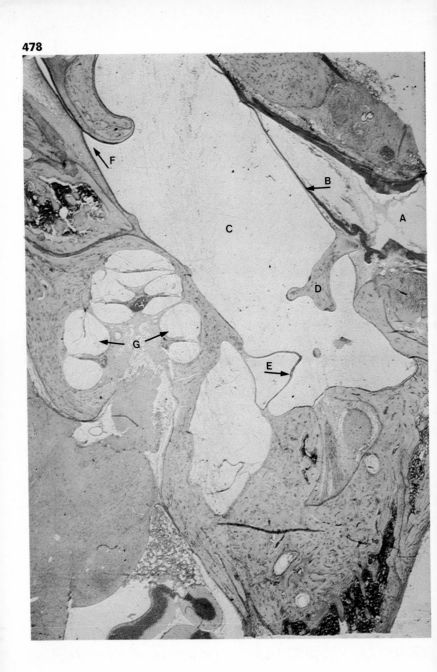

276

478 *External, middle and inner ear (H & E)* This section through the petrous portion of the temporal bone of a kitten shows:

A, external auditory meatus
B, tympanic membrane
C, cavity of middle ear
D, malleus
E, stapes
F, eustachian tube
G, cochlea

479 *Middle ear (H & E)* The handle of the malleus (A) and tympanic membrane (B) from **478** under medium power. The cavities of external auditory meatus (C) and middle ear (D) flank the ear drum.

480 *Middle ear (H & E)* High power of **479** to show the tympanic membrane. It is covered externally by epidermis (A) and internally by the simple cubical lining epithelium (B) of the middle ear cavity. The core is of loose connective tissue.

479

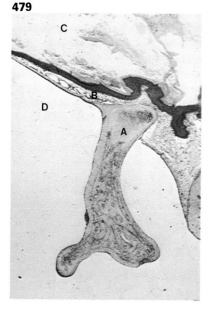

480

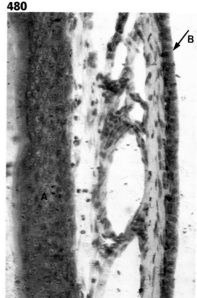

481 *Middle ear (H & E)* High power of **478** to show the stapes (A), the foot plate of which separates the cavity of the middle ear (B) from the perilymph in the vestibule (C). The footplate is fixed in the oval window by an annular fibrous joint (D).

482 *Middle ear (H & E)* High power of **478** to show the opening of the eustachian tube (A) into the cavity of the middle ear (B).

483 *Eustachian tube (H & E)* A transverse section through the cartilaginous part of the tube is shown. The cartilage (A) is hook-shaped and hyaline in type. Mucous salivary glands lie at B.

484 *Eustachian tube (H & E)* High power of **478** to show the bony part of the tube. Compact bone (A) occupies most of the field. The lining epithelium is pseudo-stratified columnar with goblet cells.

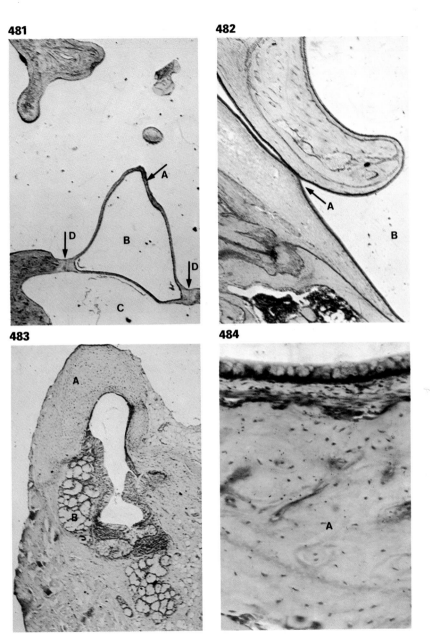

279

485 *Inner ear (H & E)* A section through the ampulla of a semicircular canal. The wall of the bony semicircular canal (A) is of compact bone. The membranous semicircular canal (B) contains a crista (C). A branch of the vestibular nerve lies at D.

486 *Inner ear, crista (H & E)* High power of the crista from **485**. The epithelial covering is tall columnar and contains hair cells and sustentacular cells. At the base of the crista the epithelium becomes cubical. The cupula is arrowed.

487 *Inner ear, macula (H & E)* Part of the bony wall of the vestibule is shown (A). Within the vestibule lies either the utricle or the saccule, the thin wall of which lies at B. A macula lies at C.

488 *Inner ear, macula (H & E)* High power of **487** to show the edge of the macula and continuity of the simple squamous epithelium of the rest of the membranous labyrinth (A) with the columnar epithelium of the macula (B).

489 *Inner ear, macula (H & E)* High power of **487** to show the macula. The otolithic membrane (A) overlies the tall columnar epithelium of the macula.

485

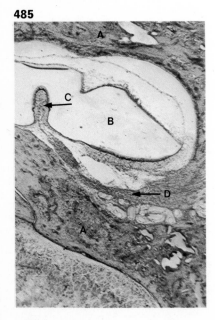

486

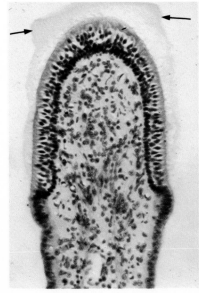

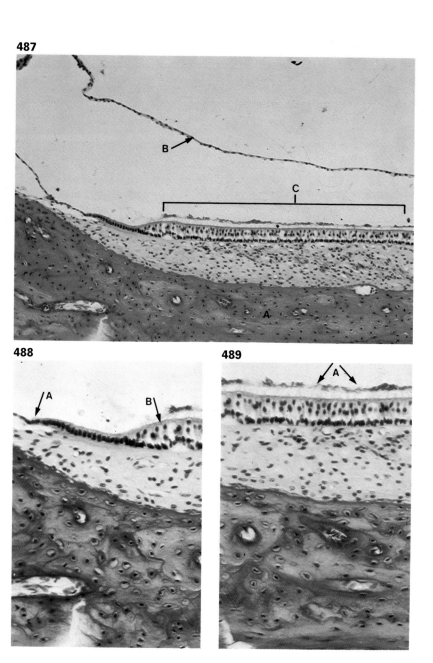

490 *Inner ear, cochlea (H & E)* The walls of the bony cochlea are of compact bone. The membranous labyrinth, lined by epithelium, is arrowed. The scala vestibuli (A) and scala tympani (B) are lined by endothelium and full of perilymph. The vestibular membrane (of Reissner) (C) is composed of a layer of endothelium and a layer of squamous epithelium.

491 *Inner ear, cochlea (H & E)* High power of **490** to show the vestibular membrane (A), stria vascularis (B), spiral ligament (C), and basilar membrane (D).

492 *Inner ear, organ of Corti (H & E)* The key to the lettering is as follows: A, osseous spiral lamina. B, spiral ganglion. C, vestibular membrane. D, tectorial membrane. E, basilar membrane. F, spiral ligament.

493 *Inner ear, organ of Corti (H & E)* The key to the lettering is as follows: A, inner hair cell. B, outer hair cells. C, inner pillar. D, inner tunnel. E, outer pillar. F, tectorial membrane.

490

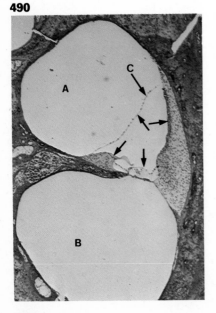

491

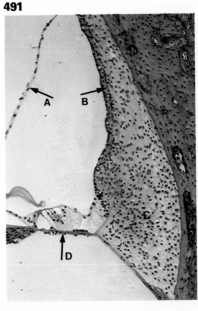

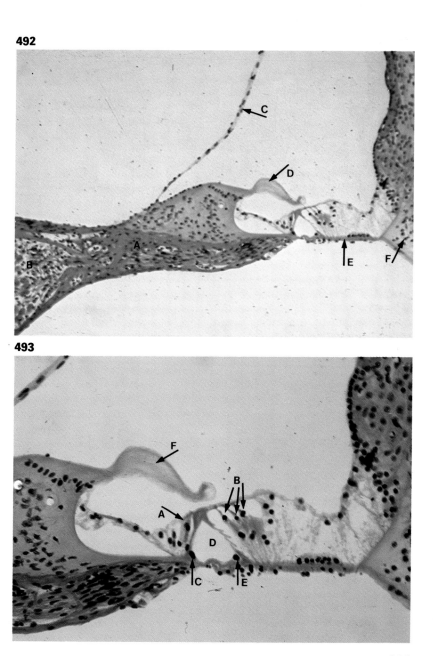

The Visual Apparatus

THE EYELID

The eyelid is covered externally by thin lax skin containing fine hairs and small sebaceous and sweat glands. It is covered internally by the conjunctiva, a typical mucous membrane composed of stratified columnar epithelium resting on loose connective tissue. Around the free margin of the eyelid the epidermis gives way to stratified squamous epithelium of mucous membrane type which gives way in turn to the conjunctival epithelium.

The core of the eyelid posteriorly contains the tarsal plate, a layer of dense connective tissue, to which the conjunctival mucosa is firmly attached. In front of this lies the skeletal muscle of the orbicularis oculi. Near the free margin of the eyelid are the large hair follicles (devoid of arrectores pilorum muscles) which give rise to the eyelashes. Also here are typical large sebaceous glands (of Meibom) which have a large duct lined by stratified squamous epithelium of mucous membrane variety. Some modified 'apocrine' sweat glands (of Moll) are also found. The sebaceous glands associated with the eyelashes are the glands of Zeis.

THE LACRIMAL GLAND

There is a compound tubulo-alveolar salivary gland of pure serous type which opens into the conjunctival sac by means of about a dozen ducts lined by simple or stratified cubical epithelium. The alveoli are lined by truncated pyramidal cells which may contain apical secretory granules. Myoepithelial cells are present. The interlobular connective tissue contains large nerves, and many lymphocytes and plasma cells.

THE FIBROUS COAT OF THE EYEBALL

The cornea

This avascular tissue exhibits five layers from without inwards. Anteriorly is stratified squamous epithelium of mucous membrane variety resting on a highly developed basement membrane (of Bowman). The bulk of the cornea is made up of the substantia propria corneae which is composed of collagenous lamellae the fibres of which in any given lamella run parallel but the fibres in adjacent lamellae run in different directions. Between the lamellae lie highly branched modified fibroblasts (corneal corpuscles) whose slender branching processes make contact with those of their neighbours. The fourth layer is a highly refractile homogeneous membrane (of Descemet) rich in elastic tissue. Finally, the endothelium of the superficial wall of the anterior chamber of the eye lies in contact with the deep aspect of the cornea. At the margins of the cornea the epithelium changes to the stratified columnar epithelium of the conjunctiva.

The sclera

Unlike the cornea which is translucent, the sclera is opaque. The sclera is composed of dense, regular connective tissue consisting of collagenous bundles separated by highly elastic areolar connective tissue with many fibroblasts. Blood vessels are found in the sclera. The tendons of the extrinsic ocular muscles are inserted into the sclera. Pigmented connective tissue cells occur in the sclera at the following sites: near the exit of the optic nerve, at the corneo-sclerotic junction, and in the lamina fusca, the inner layer of the sclera. Lymph spaces separate the lamina fusca from the middle coat of the eyeball, the choroid.

THE VASCULAR COAT OF THE EYEBALL

The choroid

The choroid is composed of three layers from without inwards:
The lamina suprachoroidea. This is a film of loose connective tissue containing large highly branched chromatophores.
A middle vascular layer. This is composed of loose connective tissue, and in its outer portion contains large blood vessels and pigmented connective tissue cells whilst the inner part is non-pigmented and contains a capillary network.
The lamina vitrea. An inner thin translucent homogeneous membrane.

The ciliary body

The ciliary body is a localised expansion of the vascular coat. It consists of smooth muscle embedded in pigmented loose connective tissue. The smooth muscle is arranged in inner circular, middle radial and outer meridional layers. The ciliary processes have a core of pigmented loose connective tissue and are covered by lamina vitrea and the two-layered pars ciliaris retinae which is arranged in such fashion as to bear a high resemblance to a stratified columnar epithelium, the deep layer of which is highly pigmented: the blind part of the retina is invaginated into the ciliary body in places, giving the appearance of glands.

The iris

The iris has a core of loose connective tissue containing stellate pigmented connective tissue cells. It is covered anteriorly by the endothelium of the posterior wall of the anterior chamber of the eye. Behind, it is covered by the two-layered pars iridica retinae, the inner layer of which is composed of cubical cells so packed with pigment that their outlines are lost.

The core of the iris contains smooth muscle in two places. Near the pupillary margin is circular smooth muscle (sphincter pupillae) and further peripherally and near the posterior surface of the iris is radially arranged smooth muscle (dilator pupillae). Near the base of the iris is a circle of large arteries.

The lens

The lens is a transparent ovoid located between the anterior and posterior chambers of the eye. It is composed of a capsule, an anterior epithelium and lens fibres.

The capsule of the lens is a highly elastic membrane. The anterior lens epithelium is simple cubical. The lens fibres make up the substance of the lens. They are elongated prisms arranged meridionally in lamellae. The oldest fibres lie posteriorly and are anucleate.

THE NERVOUS COAT OF THE EYEBALL

The retina

The retina is an outlying part of the central nervous system: it has no regenerative powers therefore and has neuroglia as its supporting tissue. It is arranged in a ten-layered visual part posteriorly and a two-layered blind portion anteriorly. The junction from one to the other is gradual and resembles a flight of steps: it is known as the ora serrata. The blind portion of the retina is applied to the inner aspect of the iris and ciliary body and has been described already.

Three neurones are involved in transmitting the impulse across the visual portion of the retina, which possesses ten layers from without inwards, as follows:

1. The pigmented layer. This consists of a single layer of hexagonal pigmented cells next to the choroid. Each cell is related to about a dozen rods and cones and extrudes fine processes of pigmented cytoplasm between them.

2. The rods and cones. This layer is composed of the non-nucleated portions of the rods and cones which are cylinders or cones as the case may be, and which are modified dendrites. Both are rich in mitochondria and their outer parts are seen with the E.M. to be modified cilia.

3. The outer limiting membrane. The expanded outer extremity of neuroglial cells known as fibres of Müller forms with its fellows a discontinuous layer at the junction between the nucleated and non-nucleated portions of the rods and cones, and is known as the outer limiting membrane. The Müller fibres form junctional complexes with the rods and cones.

4. The nuclei of the rods and cones. This zone is composed of some five or six rows of nuclei. The oval cone nuclei form the outermost row and inside this are several rows of circular rod nuclei.

5. The outer synaptic zone. This is a homogeneous pink zone in H & E preparations. After silver staining synaptic connections between the inner rod and cone segments (axons) and the dendrites of bipolar ganglion cells are seen.

6. The bipolar ganglion cell nuclei. This zone comprises fewer rows than the nuclei of the rods and cones. It consists of the nuclei of the bipolar ganglion cells for the most part. Other neurones known as horizontal cells also lie in this layer, as well as the nucleated portion of the fibre of Müller.

7. The inner synaptic zone. Synapses occur here between the axons of the bipolar ganglion cells and the dendrites of the optic nerve cells. The layer is homogeneous, however, in H & E preparations.

8. The optic nerve cells. These are multipolar ganglion cells of a wide variety of size and they form a discontinuous layer, except near the fovea where several rows may be seen.

9. The optic nerve fibres. These are the non-myelinated axons of the optic nerve cells.

10. The inner limiting membrane. This layer is composed of the expanded bases of the fibres of Müller.

There are approximately ten rods for every cone in the retina. At the macula, blood vessels are absent, a yellow pigment is found and in the centre of the macula (fovea) cones alone are found and are here shaped like rods. In the fovea the inner layers of the retina are displaced to the side so that light falls directly on the photoreceptors.

The optic nerve

This 'nerve' is in reality a part of the central nervous system, as is the retina. Where the optic nerve pierces the sclera, the name *lamina cribosa* is applied. The fibres of the nerve are non-medullated up to this point, but become medullated thereafter so that the diameter of the nerve increases abruptly. The nerve is invested by dura, arachnoid and pia mater: the pia sends fine septa into the nerve substance, but it does not subdivide the single bundle of nerve fibres into fasciculi. Subdural and subarachnoid spaces surround the nerve.

The nerve substance is composed of medullated nerve fibres and neuroglial cells. In the middle lie the central artery and vein of the retina.

494 *Eyelid (H & E)* The epidermis (A) and conjunctival epithelium (B) cover the outer and inner aspects of the eyelid. Skeletal muscle lies at C and eyelashes at D. The glands of Meibom (E) and of Moll (F) are also conspicuous.

495 *Eyelid (H & E)* High power of **494** to show the sebaceous glands of Meibom and their duct (*top*).

496 *Eyelid (H & E)* High power of **494** to show the modified sweat glands (of Moll) with a lining of simple cubical epithelium. Cf. **218** and **476**.

497 *Lacrimal gland (H & E)* The gland is composed of serous acini (A). Intercalated (B) and intralobular ducts (C) also occur.

498 *Cornea (H & E)* The stratified squamous epithelium (A), substantia propria (B), membrane of Descemet (C), and endothelium (D) can be made out. The basement membrane (of Bowman) of the epithelium cannot.

499 *Cornea (Gold chloride)* The fibroblasts of the substantia propria corneae are well brought out by this method.

494

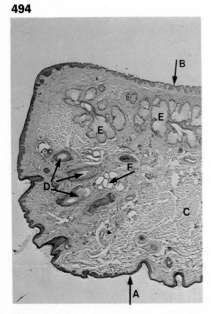

495

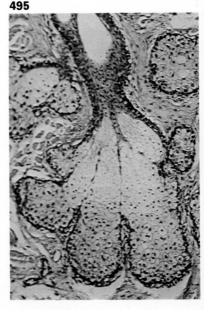

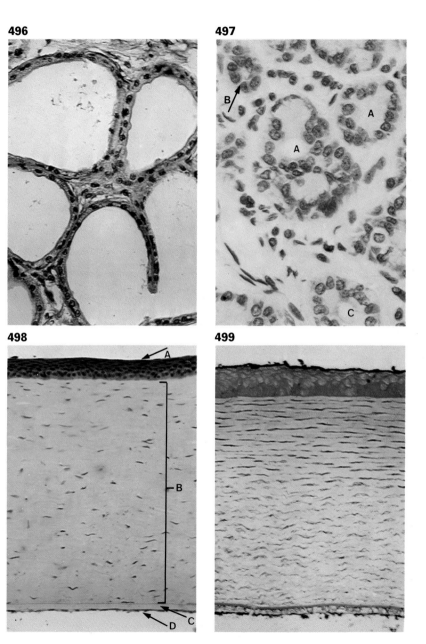

289

500 *Cornea (Gold chloride)* The lamellae of the substantia propria corneae are clearly seen in this preparation.

501 *Cornea (Gold chloride)* The stellate fibroblasts of the corneal substantia propria are delineated in this preparation.

502 *Corneo-sclerotic junction (H & E)* The cornea (A), sclera (B), and conjunctiva (C) are shown. The corneo-sclerotic junction (D) contains pigmented cells.

503 *Wall of eyeball (H & E)* Section of the wall of the eyeball showing retina (A), choroid (B) and sclera (C). The inferior oblique muscle (D) is here inserted into the sclera.

504 *Wall of eyeball (H & E)* The retina (A), choroid (B), and sclera (C) form the wall of the eyeball. The inferior oblique muscle (D) is here attached to the sclera, which is composed of dense connective tissue.

500
501

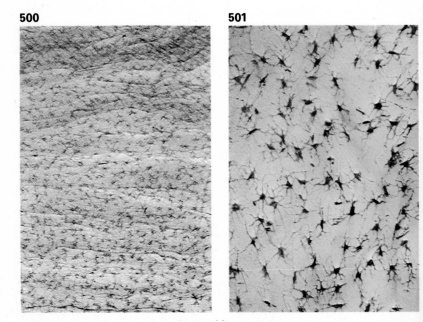

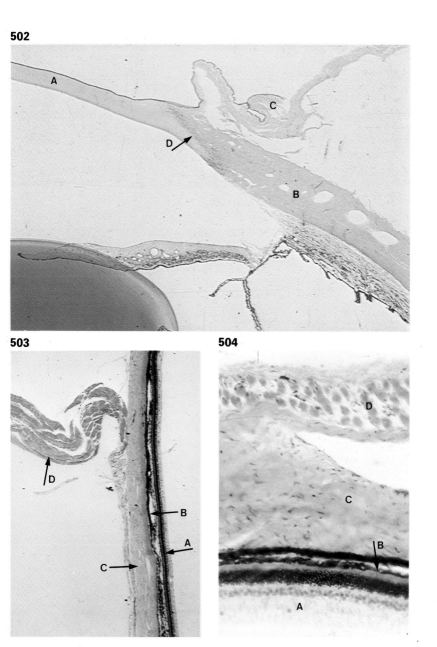

291

505 *Front of eyeball (H & E)* The plane of section is through lens (A), iris (B), ciliary body (C), and sclera (D). Ciliary processes are present at E.

506 *Iris (H & E)* The iris is covered anteriorly by endothelium (A) and posteriorly by the two-layered pars iridica retinae which is arranged in outer non-pigmented (B) and inner pigmented (C) layers. The core of the iris is composed of pigmented loose connective tissue (D).

507 *Iris (H & E)* Section near the periphery of the iris to show the smooth muscle of dilator pupillae (*arrows*).

508 *Iris (H & E)* Section near the pupillary margin to show the smooth muscle of sphincter pupillae (*arrows*).

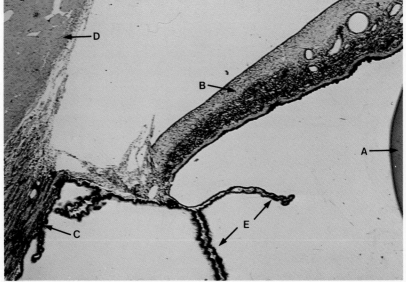

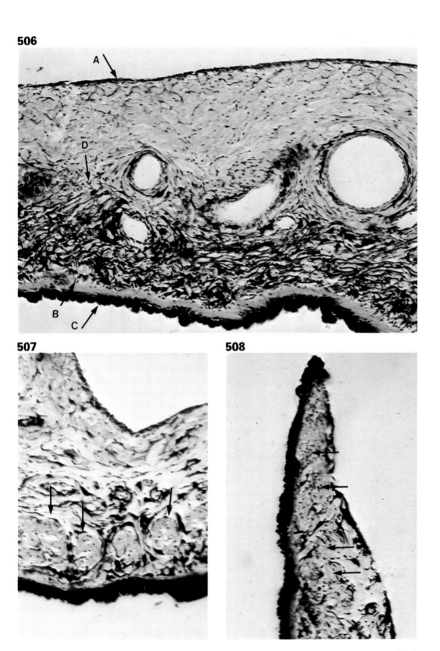

293

509 *Ciliary body (H & E)* Higher power view to show the pars ciliaris retinae arranged in outer pigmented (A) and inner non-pigmented (B) layers. The ciliary muscle stains pink.

510 *Ciliary process (H & E)* The ciliary processes have a core of pigmented loose connective tissue (A) and are covered by the two-layered pars ciliaris retina which is disposed in inner non-pigmented (B) and outer pigmented (C) layers.

511 *Lens (Azan)* Section of the developing lens to show the anterior lens epithelium (A) and the posterior lens epithelium (B) from which the lens fibres will develop.

512 *Lens (H & E)* Section through the lens equator to show continuity between the anterior lens epithelium (A) and the nucleated lens fibres (B) found here.

513 *Lens (H & E)* Section through the lens fibres which are anucleate pyramids.

509

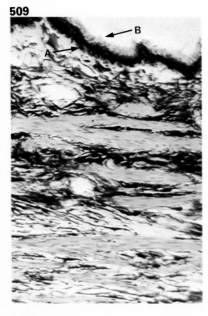

510

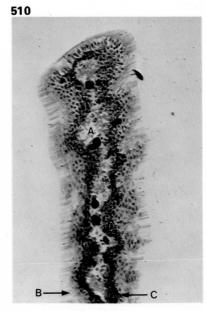

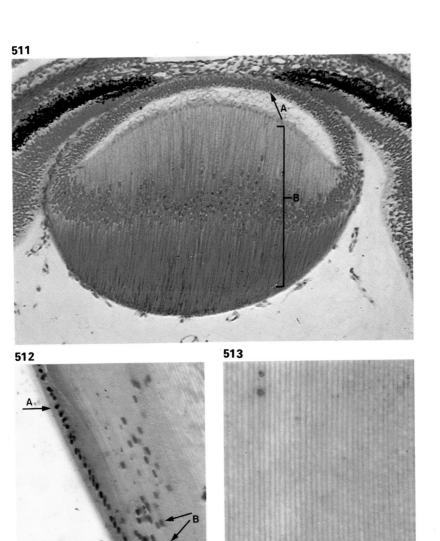

511

512

513

295

514 *Back of eyeball (H & E)* This section of human eyeball shows the retina (A), choroid (B), and sclera (C). The macula lies at D and the exit of the optic nerve (blind spot) at E.

515 *Wall of eyeball (H & E)* This field shows the retina (A), choroid (B), and sclera (C) of the human eye.

516 *Ora serrata (H & OGE)* In this field the ten-layered visual portion of the retina (A) gives way to the two-layered blind portion (B).

517 *Retina and choroid (H & E)* The retina at low power shows eight distinct layers, of which the outermost is the pigmented layer (A). The rods and cones (B) lie in the outermost part of the retina and light has to penetrate the inner layers to reach the photoreceptors.

514

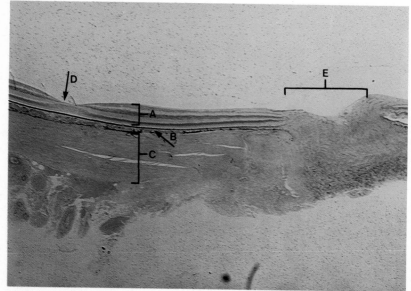

515

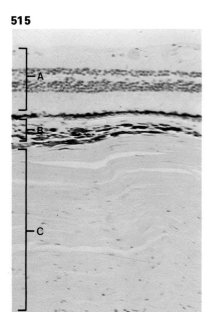

516

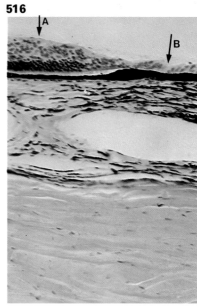

517

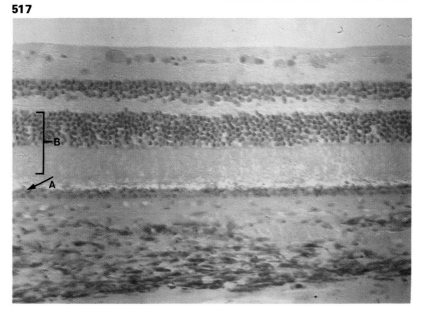

518 *Retina, fovea centralis (H & E)* In contrast to the situation obtaining elsewhere in the retina the photoreceptors at the fovea (*arrows*) are exposed directly to the light impulse because the inner layers of the retina are not represented here.

519 *Retina (H & E)* Eight of the ten layers of typical retina are obvious here. The inner and outer limiting membranes are not.

    A, pigment layer
    B, rods and cones
    C, nuclei of rods and cones
    D, outer synaptic layer
    E, bipolar ganglion cell nuclei
    F, inner synaptic layer
    G, optic nerve cells
    H, optic nerve fibres

518

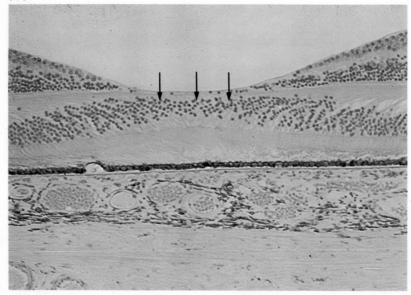

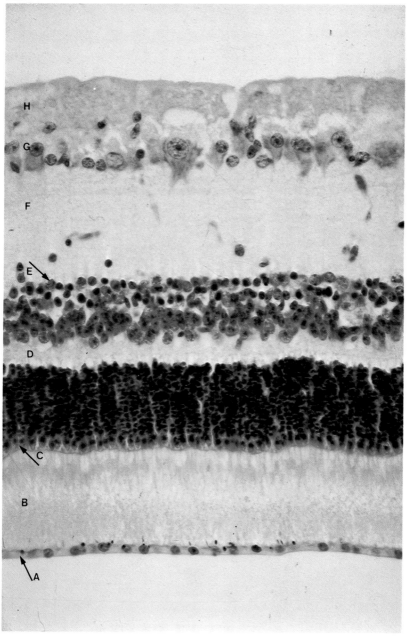

520 *Retina (Silver)* In this preparation from cat retina, the formation of the inner limiting membrane by the expanded inner extremity of the fibres of Müller is well demonstrated (*arrows*).

521 *Exit of optic nerve (H & E)* The optic nerve pierces the sclera at the lamina cribrosa (A) and at once expands as its fibres become myelinated. The arachnoid (B), and dura (C), with the subarachnoid space (D) are also seen.

522 *Exit of optic nerve (H & E)* High power of **521** to show the optic nerve fibres (A) piercing the lamina cribrosa (B) to form the optic nerve (C).

523 *TS optic nerve (H & E)* The optic nerve is a single funiculus of medullated nerve fibres and is invested by pia (A) and arachnoid (B) with the subarachnoid space (C) between. The pia sends fine septa into the nerve substance.

524 *Optic nerve (H & E)* High power of **523** to show pial septa (A), medullated nerve fibres (B), and neuroglial nuclei (C).

520

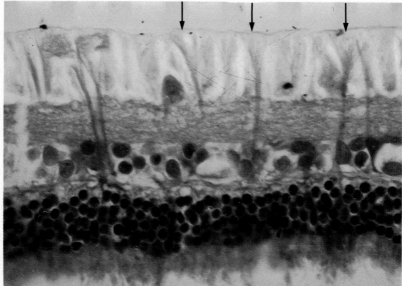

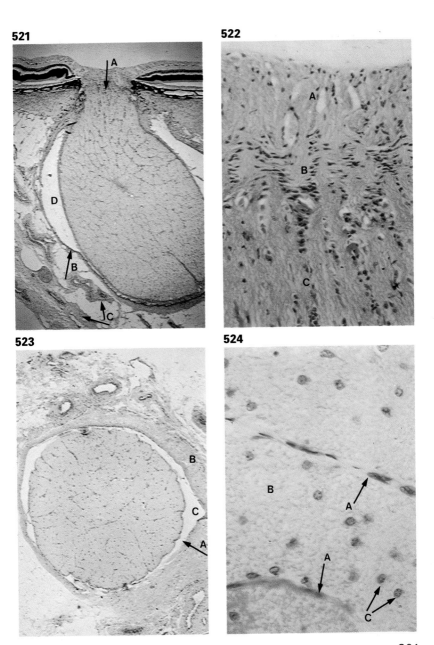

521

522

523

524

The Olfactory Apparatus

The olfactory mucosa is of yellow colour, unlike the rest of the nasal mucosa which is bright red. The olfactory epithelium is found in the roof of the nasal cavity, on the upper part of the nasal septum and on the superior nasal concha. The epithelium is pseudo-stratified ciliated columnar and contains nerve cells supported by epithelial cells of two types, basal and supporting. Many rows of nuclei occur. Next to the surface is a single row of oval nuclei belonging to the supporting cells. Deep to this are many rows of round nuclei of the olfactory nerve cells, and the basal cells.

The olfactory cells
These are bipolar ganglion cells. The round nucleus is deeply placed in the cell. The apical portion of the cell is a modified dendrite and extends to the surface where it ends in a bulbous expansion from which about half a dozen non-motile cilia arise. The base of the cell tapers rapidly to form an axon, which is unmyelinated. It passes into the underlying connective tissue, and joins its fellows to form the olfactory nerve bundles.

The supporting cells
These cells are tall columns with a single oval nucleus near the surface. They have many microvilli at their free surface and form junctional complexes, as seen with the E.M., with the adjacent olfactory neurones. Their cytoplasm contains pigment granules that impart the yellow colour to the olfactory region.

The basal cells
These triangular entities stain deeply. They lie between the bases of the other cells.

The olfactory epithelium lacks a basement membrane. The lamina propria deep to the epithelium contains many vascular capillaries as well as lymphatic capillaries. Here are also found compound tubulo-alveolar serous salivary glands (of Bowman) and some 20 fila olfactoria. The deepest part of the lamina propria contains a plexus of large veins.

525 *Nasal cavity (H & E)* Preparation from a kitten showing the nasal
septum (A) and conchae (B). Both are covered by the ciliated columnar
epithelium of the upper respiratory tract (C) and by olfactory epithelium (D).

525

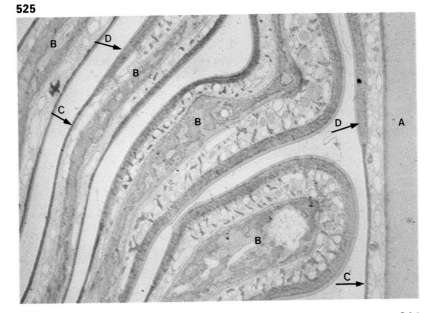

526 *Olfactory mucosa (H & E)* High power of **525** to show the olfactory epithelium (A), and nerve (B), glands of Bowman (C), blood vessels (D), and bone (E).

527 *Olfactory mucosa (H & E)* Human olfactory epithelium showing oval sustentacular nuclei (A), and round olfactory cell nuclei (B), with glands of Bowman (C) and their ducts (D). An olfactory nerve bundle lies at E.

526

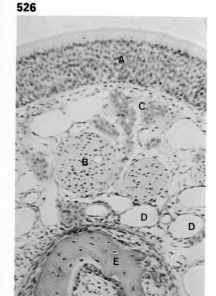

527

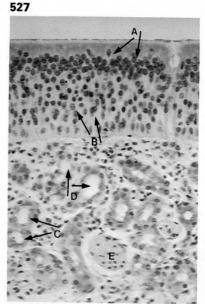

Bone Development

Bone develops in mesenchyme (primitive connective tissue). It may do so in one of two ways. The mesenchyme may elaborate in hyaline cartilage a model of the bone which is transformed subsequently into bone: this is called intracartilaginous (endochondral) ossification. Alternatively the mesenchyme may transform into bone directly, which process is known as intramembranous ossification. Newly-formed bone is invariably cancellous in nature, whether created in membrane or in cartilage.

Ossification in membrane

Mesenchyme is a composite of primitive connective cells lying in a matrix of amorphous ground substance containing immature collagen fibres. The undifferentiated mesenchymal cells transform into osteoblasts (bone forming cells) which have a basophilic cytoplasm, and they synthesise osteoid (inorganic bone matrix) which is deposited around the cells. In the process the osteoid from adjacent cells merges and some of the osteoblasts come to be surrounded on all sides by bone matrix: they are thereafter known as osteocytes or bone cells. The spicules of bone formed in this way are augmented by the activity of osteoblasts at the surface of the spicule. The immature collagen fibres become incorporated in the osteoid. Later the osteoid becomes calcified to form primary bone. Around the periphery of the primary bone eosinophilic multinucleate giant cells known as osteoclasts make their appearance. They too are derived from undifferentiated mesenchymal cells, and are responsible for the destruction of primary bone. The form assumed by any bone is determined by the appositional growth of the osteoblasts and the resorption by the osteoclasts on its surfaces. The mesenchyme condenses around the focus of primary bone to form the periosteum, which soon shows ill-defined outer fibrous and inner cellular layers. The latter retains primitive connective tissue cells which may, on suitable stimulation, acquire osteogenic properties—i.e. they transform into osteoblasts.

Endochondral ossification

Here the cells of the mesenchyme differentiate into cartilage-forming cells (chondroblasts) which construct a model of the bone in hyaline cartilage. Mesenchyme condenses around the model to form a perichondrium. Growth of the cartilage model is brought about by the interstitial growth of the cartilage cells (chondrocytes) in its substance.

A primary centre of ossification occurs in the centre of the shaft of all cartilaginous bones in the seventh or eighth week of intra-uterine life. One or more secondary centres of ossification appear at each extremity of the bone at or after birth. The first sign of the primary centre of ossification is degeneration of the cartilage cells in the core of the model. The periosteum then invades the cavity so created. It carries in blood vessels and osteogenetic cells: these become osteoblasts which form a lining to the cavity and deposit osteoid on the cartilage matrix, which later becomes calcified to form primary bone. The periosteum forms a collar of bone round the primary ossification centre: this bone however is formed in membrane. With its appearance, the need for any quantity of bone in the centre of the model is reduced and so the latter is resorbed by osteoclasts and primitive bone marrow is elaborated by the mesenchyme in the spaces so created. By birth, the shaft (diaphysis) is composed of bone filled with marrow but the extremities (epiphyses) are still cartilaginous.

One or more secondary centres form in each epiphysis at or after birth. In their manner of formation they resemble the primary ossification centres. The particles of bone derived from the individual centres fuse so that the extremities of the model become converted to a single mass of bone which remains separated, until early adult life, from the diaphyseal bone by a persistent plate of hyaline cartilage known as the epiphyseal plate (or disc). In postnatal life growth in length of the bone ensues by virtue of the interstitial growth of the cartilage cells in the disc, and growth in breadth by the appositional growth of the periosteum. One epiphyseal disc disappears around the age of 18 years and the other at about 20 years: this latter is referred to as the growing end. The disc disappears because for the first time the rate at which it is being eroded and replaced by bone on its diaphyseal aspect outstrips the rate of interstitial growth of the hyaline cartilage of the disc. When the disc has been replaced by bone the epiphysis is described as having closed.

---

528 *Intramembranous ossification (H & E)* The shafts of long bones become broader, as here, by deposition of membrane bone (A) by the osteoblasts (B) of the periosteum (C).

529 *Intramembranous ossification (H & E)* High power of **528** to show a seam of osteoblasts (A) depositing bone (B) with trapped osteoblasts (C) becoming bone cells. Two osteoclasts (D) have produced shallow erosions of the bony spicule E.

530 *Intramembranous ossification (H & OGE)* Forming mandible (A) with a seam of basophilic osteoblasts on one edge (B) and two osteoclasts (C) on the other.

531 *Intramembranous ossification (H & OGE)* As **530**, showing six eosinophilic osteoclasts (*arrows*) resorbing the mandibular bone. They are multinucleate giant cells.

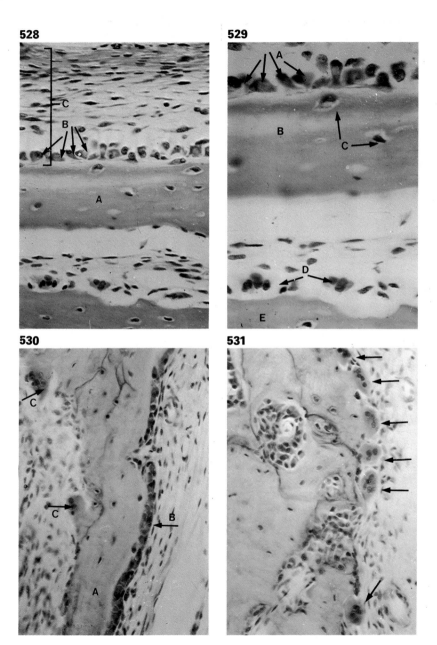

307

532 *Endochondral ossification (H & E)* A primary centre of ossification is forming in the centre of the model of hyaline cartilage. A periosteal bud (A) is extending in towards the region of degenerating cartilage cells.

533 *Endochondral ossification (H & E)* Ossification is now advanced in this primary centre in a human metatarsal. The bone is darkly stained (A). Periosteal bone (B) is forming around the centre. Hyaline cartilage lies at C.

534 *Endochondral ossification (H & E)* Even more advanced development of a primary centre of ossification than in **533**. Hyaline cartilage is at A.

535 *Endochondral ossification (H & E)* The shaft (diaphysis) is now ossified completely. The epiphysis is still cartilaginous. The metaphysis (*arrowed*) is shown under high power in the next picture.

536 *Endochondral ossification (H & E)* The zones of maturation (A) and of degeneration (B) of the epiphyseal cartilage are seen. In the metaphysis are osteoblasts (C), osteoclasts (D), and spicules of osteoid (E).

537 *Endochondral ossification (H & E)* The secondary centre of ossification has now formed in the epiphysis (A) which is bony. Cartilage persists as the epiphyseal plate (B) and as the articular cartilage (C).

532

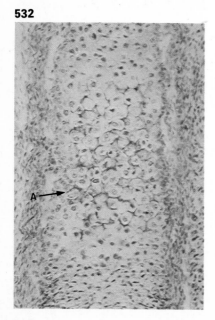

533

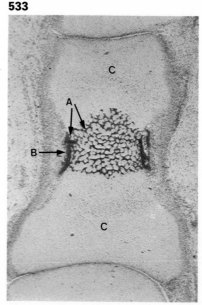

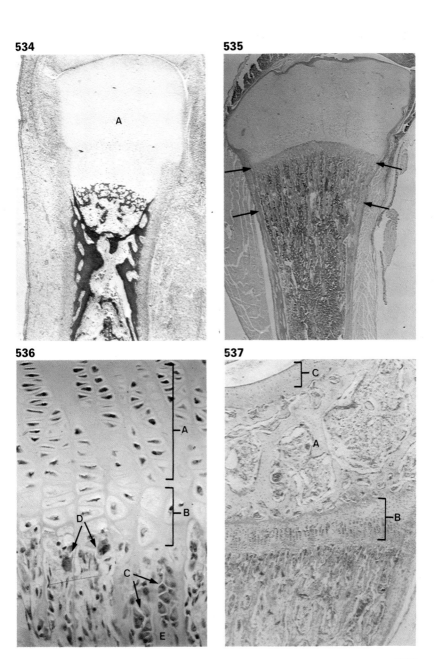

538 *Endochondral ossification (H & E)* Human elbow joint in which the epiphyses of both humerus (A) and ulna (B) have closed. Cartilage persists only over the articular surfaces (*arrows*).

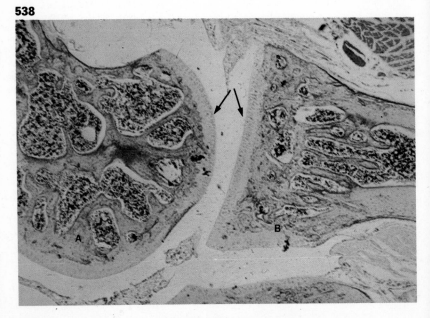

538

Tooth Development

The teeth develop intially from u-shaped thickenings—the dental laminae—of the stratified squamous epithelium of the roof and floor of the ectodermal portion of the mouth cavity. Each lamina gives rise to the appropriate number of thickenings, known as enamel organs. These project into the underlying primitive connective tissue (mesenchyme), becoming indented from below by the mesenchyme in the process, so that they become cup-shaped. The enamel organs then become detached from the overlying epithelium and so come to lie free in the mesenchyme.

Proliferation of the epithelial cells of the enamel organ causes it to become multi-layered. The superficial cells are cubical and constitute the covering layer. The superficial cells in the concavity of the cup are columnar and are known as ameloblasts since they will elaborate the enamel of the tooth. Internal to the ameloblasts are several rows of flattened cells, the stratum intermedium. The region between the stratum intermedium and the covering layer is occupied by a network of stellate epithelial cells separated by wide tracts of amorphous ground substance: this region of atypical (or reticulated) epithelium is called the stellate reticulum.

The concavity of the cup is occupied by mesenchyme known as the dental papilla. The ameloblasts lining the concavity of the cup *induce* the adjacent connective tissue cells of the dental papilla to transform into odontoblasts which will elaborate the dentine of the crown. The odontoblasts are elongated cylinders and line up side by side. At the rim of the cup the ameloblasts are continuous with the covering layer. Proliferation of the epithelial cells of the cup rim causes it to advance so that the cup becomes deeper. The advancing rim is known as Hertwig's epithelial root sheath, the cells of which induce the formation of more odontoblasts from the mesenchyme. When these odontoblasts have appeared the epithelial root sheath breaks up and disappears, leaving a column of odontoblasts which will form the dentine of the root.

Enamel is formed intra-cellularly. The ameloblasts are hexagonal on cross-section and their basal cytoplasm becomes converted into a prism of enamel which will also be of hexagonal outline therefore. The enamel becomes calcified later. The apical living portion of the ameloblast persists until the tooth erupts, after which it is rapidly removed by attrition.

Dentine is an extra-cellular compound. It is laid down by the odontoblasts near their apices (i.e. next to the basement membrane which separates them from the ameloblasts). The apical portions of the cells become reduced, as a result, to a narrow cytoplasmic thread. These threads are known as the fibres of Tomes, and run in canals in the dentine known as dentinal tubules. When first formed dentine is uncalcified and is called pre-dentine.

The cementum is produced by mesenchymal cells lying external to the odontoblasts forming the dentine of the root. Dentine is acellular near the crown of the tooth but in the deep part of the root contains stellate cells. The collagenous fibres in the proximity of the root of the tooth become embedded at one extremity in the developing bone of the jaw and at the other in the cementum. They constitute the periodontal membrane which holds the tooth anchored in its socket.

The roots of deciduous teeth become subjected to pressure from the enlarging permanent teeth, and resorption occurs. This is brought about by multinucleate giant cells called odontoclasts.

---

539 *Developing tooth (H & E)* A very early enamel organ forming in the dental lamina, a U-shaped thickening of the stratified squamous epithelium of the mouth.

540 *Developing tooth (H & E)* A later stage of development of an enamel organ. The surrounding mesenchyme is condensing. The centre of the enamel organ contains stellate reticulum (A) and the concave aspect is thickening to form ameloblasts.

541 *Developing tooth (H & E)* The enamel organ now has covering layer (A), stellate reticulum (B), and ameloblasts (C). The connective tissue papilla (D) is elaborating odontoblasts (E).

539

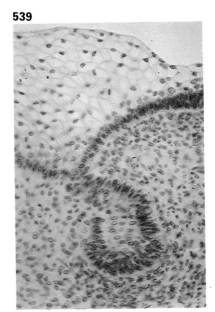

540

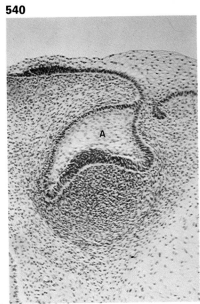

541

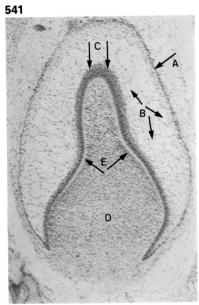

542 *Developing tooth (H & E)* The odontoblasts of the dental papilla are now obvious (A) and the clear space (B) between them and the ameloblasts (C) is the first sign of enamel.

543 *Developing tooth (H & E)* The tooth germ is now at an advanced stage of development and membrane bone (*arrows*) is forming around it.

544 *Developing tooth (H & E)* Even before it has erupted, the germ of the milk tooth (A) is showing evidence of erosion at B by the pressure to which it is being subjected by the permanent tooth germ (C).

545 *Developing tooth (H & E)* High power of **544** to show the odontoclasts (A) eroding the dentine (B) of the milk tooth germ.

546 *Developing tooth (H & E)* High power of the permanent tooth germ from **544** to show enamel organ (A) and dental papilla (B).

547 *Developing tooth (H & E)* High power of **546**. The layers are: (from enamel organ) A, covering layer; B, stellate reticulum; C, stratum intermedium; D, ameloblasts; and E, enamel. (From dental papilla) F, dentine; G, predentine; H, odontoblasts; and I, pulp cavity.

542

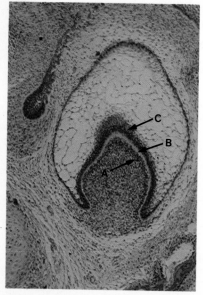

543

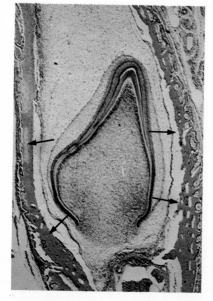

314

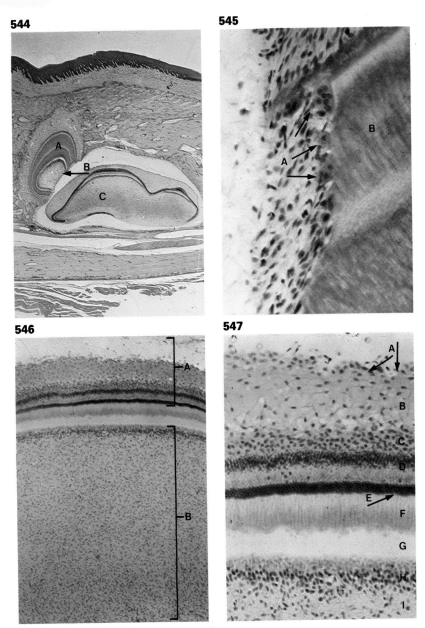

INDEX

Herring bodies, 110
Holocrine secretion, 123
Hormone(s), adrenal cortical, 107
–adrenal medullary, 107
–aldosterone, 107
–cortisol, 107
–cortisone, 107
–deoxycorticosterone, 107
–follicle-stimulating, 108
–glucagon, 151
–glucocorticoid, 107
–gonadotrophic, 108, 249
–growth, 108
–insulin, 151
–lactogenic, 108
–luteinising, 108
–melanocyte-stimulating, 108
–mineralocorticoid, 107
–oestrogenic, 249
–ovarian, 246–247
–oxytocin, 108
–parathyroid, 106
–placental, 108
–progesterone, 246, 249
–renin, 217
–testicular, 229
–testosterone, 229
–thyrocalcitonin, 106
–thyroxin, 106
–thymic, 90
–tri-iodothyronine, 106
–vasopressin, 108
Huxley's layer, 123
Hyponychium, 124, **237**
Hypophysis, alpha chromophils of, 108, **200–203**
–beta chromophils of, 108, **200–203**
–chromophobes of, 108, **200–203**
–neuro-secretion of, 108–110, **199**
–pars anterior of, 107–108
–pars intermedia of, 108
–pars nervosa of, 108–110
–pars tuberalis of, 108
–pituicytes of, 108
Ileum, 148–149, **306–308**
Integument, 120–124, **204–237**
–blood vessels of, 120, **209**
–encapsulated nerve endings of, 121, **211–213**
–glands of, 121–123, **214–224**
–nerves of, 121
Intercalated discs, 40–41, **79**
Intercellular substance, 22, 24, 26, **32, 50–52, 54–61**
Interstitial lamellae, 26, **56**
Intestine, large, 149, **309–315**
–small, 148–149, **294–308**
Intrapulmonary bronchi, 203, **356–360**
Jejunum, 148, **294–303**
Junctional complex, 9–10, 302
Keratohyalin granules, **12**
Kidney, 216–217, **365–373**
–blood vessels of, 216, **365**
–calyces of, 216
–convoluted tubules of, 216, **366–368**
–cortex of, 216, **365–370**
–glomerulus of, 216, **366, 368–370**
–juxtaglomerular apparatus of, 217, **369**
–medulla of, 216, **371–373**
–nephrons of, 216
–pyramids of, 216
Knots, syncytial, 249, **467**
Labia majora, 249, **460–461**
Labia minora, 249, **458–459**
Labyrinth, bony, 273, **490**

–membranous, 273, **485–493**
Lacteals, central of villi, **297**
Lacunae, of bone, 24–26, **55, 61**
Lamellae, of bone, 26, **56–62**
–of elastic arteries, **117–120**
Lamina propria, 9
–of ileum, **306**
–of oesophagus, **274**
–of small gut, **296**
–of tongue, **257**
Langerhans, cells of, 120, **206**
–islets of, 151, **336–337**
Larynx, 202, **343–344**
Lens, 286, **511–513**
–anterior epithelium of, 286, **511**
–capsule of, 286
–fibres of, 286, **512–513**
Leucocytes, agranular, 89
–basophil polymorphonuclear, 89, **149, 153**
–eosinophil polymorphonuclear, 89, **151–153**
–granular, 89, **148–153**
–lymphocytes, medium, 90, **147**
–lymphocytes, small, 90, **146**
–monocytes, 90, **148**
–neutrophil polymorphonuclear, 89, **150, 152–153**
Leydig, interstitial cells of, 229, **391**
Lieberkühn, crypts of, in large gut, 149, **309–310**
–in small gut, 148, **298–301**
Ligament, elastic, 22, 24, **46–49**
–spiral, of cochlea, 274, **491**
Lingual tonsil, 143
Lip, 145, **264–267**
Liver, 150, **320–327**
–bile canaliculi of, 150, **325**
–bile ducts of, 150, **324**
–cells of, 150
–lobules of, 150, **320–321**
–lymphatic vessels of, 150, **324**
–periportal canals of, 150, **324**
–reticular fibres of, 150, **327**
–sinusoids of, 150, **322–323**
–veins of, 150, **321–323**
Loop of Henle, 216, **371–373**
Lungs, 203, **356–364**
–alveolar ducts of, 203
–alveolar sacs of, 203
–alveoli of, 203, **364**
–bronchi, 203, **356–358**
–bronchioles of, 203, **361–363**
–dust cells of, 203, **362–363**
–elastic fibres of, 203, **363–364**
–pleura of, 203, **359**
Lunula of nail, 124
Lymph, 73, 92
–capillaries, 73
–lacteals, **297**
–vessels of, 73
–vessels, valves of, 73
Lymph nodes, 92, **158–167**
–afferent lymphatic of, 92, **160–161**
–capsule of, 92, **162–163**
–cortex of, 92, **158–159**
–efferent lymphatic of, 91
–germinal centres of, 92, **164–165**
–hilum of, 92
–lymphocytes of, 91–92, **162–165**
–lymphopoiesis of, 92
–macrophages of, 91–92, **162–163, 166–167**
–medulla of, 91–92, **158–159, 166–167**
–medullary cords of, **166–167**
–plasma cells of, 92
–nodules of, 92, 164–165
–paracortex of, 92, **158–159**

–reticular fibres of, 92,
–reticulo-endothelial cells of, 92, **162–163, 166–167**
–sinuses of, 92, **162–163, 166–167**
–subcapsular sinus of, 92, **162–163**
–trabeculae of, 92
Lymphocytes, of blood, 87, **146–147**
–of lymph nodes, 91–92, **162–167**
–of spleen, 92, **172–175**
–of thymus, 90, **157**
Lymphomyeloid complex, 87–92, **146–179**
Macrophages, fixed, 91, 92, **162–163, 167, 170, 326**
–free, 23, 203, **362–363**
Macula, of retina, 286, **514**
–of saccule, 273, **489**
–of utricle, 273, **489**
Malleus, 272, **478**
Mallory-Azan stain, 6
Marrow, bone, red, 89, **154–155**
–yellow, 89, **54**
Matrix, of areolar tissue, 22, **32**
–of bone, 24, **54–61**
–of cartilage, 24, **50–52**
Meatus, external auditory, 272, **474–477**
Mediastinum testis, 228
Medullary cords, **166–167**
Megakaryocytes, 90
Melanin, 120
Melanoblasts, 120
Membrane, basement, 9, **18, 19**
–basilar, 274, **491–492**
–Bowman's, 284, **498**
–Descemet's, 284, **498**
–limiting inner, of retina, 287, **520**
–limiting outer, of retina, 286
–mucous, 9
–otolithic, 273, **489**
–periodontal, 141, **239–241**
–tectorial, **492–493**
–tympanic, 272, **478–479**
–vestibular, **490**
Menstrual, cycle, 248
–phase, 248, **438**
Metamyelocytes, 89
Microglia, 55
Microphages, 88
Microvilli, 9, 148, **296**
Monoblasts, 89
Monocytes, 87
Motor end plate, 40, **72–73**
Mucosa, 9
Müller, fibres of, 286–287, **520**
Muscular tissue, 38–42, **64–83**
Musculo-tendinous junction, 74
Muscle fibres, cardiac, 38, 40–42, **77–83**
–intercalated discs of, 40–41, **79**
–lipofuscin in, 42
–myofibrils of, 40
–Purkinje fibres of, 42, **80–83**
Muscle fibres, skeletal, 38–40, **68–76**
–A bands of, 39–40, **68–70**
–actin myofilaments of, 40
–areas of Cohnheim of, 39
–dark bands of, 39, **68–70**
–endomysium of, 39, **70**
–epimysium of, 40
–H lines of, 39
–I bands of, 39–40, **68–70**
–innervation of, 40, **72–73, 75–76**
–light bands of, 39, **68–70**
–motor end plates of, 40, **72–73**
–muscle spindles of, 40, **75–76**